Tibetan medicine series

FIRST INTERNATIONAL CONFERENCE

OF TIBETAN MEDICINE

MAN – MEDICINE – SOCIETY

VENICE, April 1983
ARCIDOSSO, May 1983

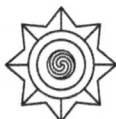

ཨོ་རྒྱན་ཆོས་འཕྲུལ་བྱ་ཀླུ་འབྱམས།

SHANG SHUNG PUBLICATIONS

This publication contains the transcription of the proceedings of the First International Conference of Tibetan Medicine held April 26–30, 1983, in the
Giorgio Cini Foundation, Venice
and the Municipality of Arcidosso, Merigar, Italy.

ORGANIZED BY THE MEDICAL CENTER OF APPLIED
PSYCHOLOGY IN VENICE,
AND THE DZOGCHEN COMMUNITY

Cover design: Yuchen Namkhai
Photos: A. Humeres, C. Ramos, L. Vitiello
Original graphics: Chögyal Namkhai Norbu
Translation from Italian: Paola Zamperini

© 2018 Shang Shung Foundation
Published by Shang Shung Publications,
an imprint of the Shang Shung Foundation
Merigar, 58031 Arcidosso (GR)
http://shop.shangshungfoundation.com
publications@shangshunginstitute.org

ISBN: 978-88-7834-162-3

This publication is the result of the selfless work of many members of the International Dzogchen Community Heartfelt thanks to all these collaborators

Special thanks to our Teacher Chögyal Namkhai Norbu

List of Topics

1. Health and Disease
2. Types of Diagnosis
3. Therapies
4. Pharmacopoeia
5. Doctor Training
6. Astrology and Medicine
7. Obstetrics, Gynecology, and Pediatrics
8. Spiritual Practices and Medicine
9. Yantra Yoga and Medicine
10. Psychology: The Nature of Mind
11. Tibetan Medicine in the West
12. Nature of Mind
13. Psychiatry: Understandings of Mental Illness

ROUNDTABLES with the participation of professors and Tibetan and European doctors on:

1. The Concept of Mind, and the Relationship between Body, Energy, and Mind
2. Understandings of Illness

Table of Contents

Introduction: Gino Vitiello   15

Preface   19

PRESENTATIONS IN VENICE

Tuesday, April 26, 1983

Moderator: Architect Paolo Rosa Salva

1. Inaugural Speech: Opening speech by local authorities   29

2. Professor Namkhai Norbu: Introduction to Tibetan medicine 40

Origins and sources of Tibetan Medicine. Person as a totality of body, voice or energy, and mind. Energy and its importance in a person's well-being. Illness and health: the three humors. Classifications of diseases, including those induced by external provocation, and karmic, accidental, trauma-induced sickness, and life illnesses. Mantra and medicine. Karma is not unavoidable. Mind and its influence on the body. Healing methods: medicines, therapies, behavior, and diet. Medicine and Astrology. Medicine and Yantra Yoga. Medicine and Tantrism. Eastern and Western Medicine.

3. Doctor Tsarong Jigme Tsewang: Fundamental Principles of Tibetan medicine   54

Medicine and Buddhism. The three vital processes. Mind and matter. Composition of medications. Therapies, diet, and life style. The eight branches of Tibetan medicine. Diagnostic methods.

4. **Doctor Trogawa Rinpoche: History of Tibetan medicine. Medicine and Dharma**   70

History of Tibetan medicine: the origins. Developments, fourth century: Biji Kaje; seventh Century: First International Gathering; eighth century: Second International Gathering. The translator Berotsana. Eleventh century: Trapa Ngönshe and the rediscovery of medical texts. Twentieth century: founding of the Tibetan Medical College in Lhasa. Family lineages. Medicine and Dharma: the physician's deontology. Passions, humors, and sickness.

WEDNESDAY, APRIL 27, 1983

MODERATOR: DOCTOR TSARONG JIGME TSEWANG

5 **Doctor Lobsang Drolma: Obstetrics and gynecology in Tibetan medicine**   78

The three types of women. The menstrual cycle. Conception and related emotions. The four types of consciousness that are reborn. Embryonic development. The five elements and the physical body. Consciousness and the five sense organs. Formation of winds. Birth.

6. **Doctor Trogawa Rinpoche: Pulse Diagnosis, Part I**   84

Diagnostics: the exam of the pulse and the thirteen factors to consider: 1. the preliminaries; 2. the time; 3. the point; 4. the pressure to exert; 5. the interpretation of information gathered; 6. the natural condition of the pulse; 7. the pulse and the seasons: the five elements and the four relations.
8. The seven wondrous pulses (a. the condition of one's home; b. forecast on travels and guests; c. war; d. business; e. negative external influences; f. substitute pulse; g. pregnancy); 9. difference between a healthy and unhealthy pulse; 10. pinpointing the disease; 11. death pulse; 12. demonic pulse;

13. the la pulse (pulse of the strength of the individual); Other diagnostic methods.

8. Professor Namkhai Norbu: Dealing with Incurable Illnesses 104

Humor imbalance as cause of sickness. Classification of illnesses: singular and conjoined (denpa): duwa and lanyen (accompanied by external provocations) dretren and lhogtren illnesses. Mantra, energy, and breathing. Medicine, astrology, and mo. Communication and collaboration with the patient. Moxabustion, acupuncture, and bloodletting.

THURSDAY, APRIL 28, 1983

Moderator: Doctor Fernand Meyer

9. Doctor Lobsang Drolma: Delivery and Post-natal Care 118

Determining the sex of the fetus. Auspicious rituals celebrated at birth. Delivery complications. Breast infections and related causes. The stages of breast cancer. Treatments. The most common female ailments.

10. Doctor Tenzin Chödrak: Astrology and Medicine 128

The seven pulse examinations. Influence of seasons and constellations on the healthy pulse. The pulse and the five elements. The pulse in a sick person. How to correctly examine the pulse. Mental illnesses.

11. Doctor Tsarong Jigme: Pharmacology and Pharmacodynamics 139

Pharmacology, proto-elements, and their combinations. The six flavors and their influence on the three humors; the benefits and the damage they bring, if taken in excess. The pharmacological ingredients.

FRIDAY, APRIL 29, 1983

Moderator: Barrie Simmons

12. Professor Barrie Simmons: Psychotherapy, Self-acceptance, and Tibetan Medicine   146

Conference as a professional and self-development opportunity. Conscious and unconscious mind. The Nature of reality. Psychotherapy and psychiatry. To awaken awareness. Self, and self-image. The Meaning of self-acceptance. Illness and health. The Symptom.

13. Professor Rakra Tethong Rinpoche: The Education of Tibetan Children in Switzerland   156

History of Tibet: the Bön tradition and its influences on Tibetan culture. The importance of Shang Shung for Tibetan science. The five elements, the five passions, the five wisdoms. The Importance of teaching Tibetan culture to the Tibetan children in Switzerland.

14. Doctor Tashi Tazan: The Tibetan Youth Association in Europe   164

15. Professor Namkhai Norbu: Medicine and Yantra Yoga   168

The meaning of yoga. Yoga and energy disturbances. Religion and Dharma. Body, speech, mind, and the nature of mind. Dualism and attachment as causes of problems. Hatha Yoga and Yantra Yoga. Re-educating breathing with the preliminary movements of Yantra Yoga. Yoga and Visualization.

SATURDAY, APRIL 30, 1983, MORNING SESSION

Moderator: Professor Giorgio Monaco

First Round Table   181

Professor Monaco, Professor Donato, Doctor Trogawa Rinpoche, Doctor Lobsang Drolma, Doctor Tenzin Chödrak, Doctor Luigi Vitiello

Sᴀᴛᴜʀᴅᴀʏ, Aᴘʀɪʟ 30, 1983, ᴀғᴛᴇʀɴᴏᴏɴ sᴇssɪᴏɴ

Moderator: Professor Barrie Simmons

Second Round Table   201

*Professor Namkhai Norbu, Doctor Tenzin Chödrak, Doctor
Carlos Ramos*

PRESENTATIONS IN ARCIDOSSO   213

Mᴏɴᴅᴀʏ, Mᴀʏ 2, 1983

Inauguration: Opening speeches by local authorities   217

Wᴇᴅɴᴇsᴅᴀʏ, Mᴀʏ 4, 1983

Doctor Trogawa Rinpoche: Mental Illness   227

Tʜᴜʀsᴅᴀʏ, Mᴀʏ 5, 1983

Doctor Tenzin Chödrak: The Nature of Mind   231

Fʀɪᴅᴀʏ, Mᴀʏ 6, 1983

Doctor Lobsang Drolma: The Nature of Mind   233

*Medicine and the teaching. Medicine and society. Request for fast
acting medicine. A complete recovery requires the collaboration
of the patient. Awareness, diet, and behavior. Medicine and
culture.*

Saturday, May 6, 1983

Professor Namkhai Norbu: Man, Medicine, and Society   235

*Medicine and the teaching. Medicine and society. Request for fast
acting medicine. A complete recovery requires the collaboration of
the patient. Awareness, diet, and behavior. Medicine and culture.*

List of Invited Speakers   245

Introduction

There are events whose significance is hard to fathom at the time of their unfolding. In 1983 Namkhai Norbu, then professor of Tibetan language and culture at the Istituto Orientale at the University of Napoli, managed to organize, with the help of a handful of students, the first international conference of Tibetan medicine in the West, by gathering the principal experts of Tibetan medicine as well as some among the most important European representatives – truly an amazing feat. Venice and Arcidosso were the locations for this conference that took places over two weeks' time.

I believe that at the time very few people were aware of the existence of Tibetan medicine. If one browses the Italian language publications related to this topic that were printed before this conference, one will find very few titles, mostly translations of English language scholarship. In the following years, however, many more works were published, both in Italy and abroad. Clearly a shift had occurred: this conference had introduced a new form of knowledge and generated a great interest.

One of the themes that emerged in those days is the need to approach Tibetan medical culture without prejudice and preconceived notions and with the open-minded curiosity that is the basis of every form of knowledge. Only in this fashion we will be able to enter in the complex mechanisms of this medical system that offers us a holistic approach, that is, a reading of human beings that is profound and rigorously logic – if we understand its premises. This approach is not limited to a mechanic and organismic vision of the human body, but one that puts forth the integration of the three fundamental aspects of our existence – body, mind, and energy – as our most advanced research has recently also begun to show us. This encounter has permanently shaped the way in which I, who was a young doctor back then, as well as other colleagues who had the good fortune to take part in it, have related to the medical profession in the years to come.

Namkhai Norbu's commitment and his research in this field are not limited to the 1983 conference: a few years later, in 1989, he founded the International Shang Shung Institute for Tibetan Studies (that later became a foundation), which organized first the Tibetan Medicine Symposium at Amherst College in 2008 (https://www.amherst.edu/system/files/styles/original/private/media/1947/Tibetan-Medicine2.jpg), and then a third international conference of Tibetan Medicine at the Rubin Museum in New York in 2014 (https://www.indiegogo.com/projects/historic-tibet-an-medicine-conference-at-the-rubin-museum-of-art#/). Since 2010, meetings and conferences on specific themes related to Tibetan medicine have been regularly held in Tenerife and Barcelona, and the International Shang Shung Institute for Tibetan Studies and the Arura Tibetan Medicine Group of Qinghai (China) signed a collaboration agreement in Tenerife in 2013. In the United States, the Tibetan Medicine School of the International Shang Shung Institute, directed by Doctor Phuntsog Wangmo, has organized a four-year course that has produced its first graduates in 2013, with a graduation ceremony held at Amherst College.

Thanks to this effort and to the ensuing result for this very ancient science, nowadays Tibetan medicine is no longer confused with its more famous relatives, as it were, namely Indian Ayurveda and Chinese medicine, and it has gone on to gain the identity and the recognition it deserves, so much so that the Chinese government plans to put forth to UNESCO its nomination as world heritage.

When, a few years ago, we began the transcription of the proceedings of the 1983 conference, it became immediately clear the task would not be simple for a variety of reasons: we had a serious challenge of translating terms and ideas that were foreign to our understanding. At times, it is hard for lay people to understand even in their own language the medical jargon doctors use to communicate among themselves. When this task involves translating concepts absent from one's cultural tradition from a foreign language that has different semantic roots, it becomes even more complex.

Each medical tradition represents a specific understanding of the human condition, and different cultures do not always resonate with each other in this regard, therefore it is really easy to fail to convey the meanings of words and ideas in the translation process. Perhaps the ones bound to have the greatest difficulty to understand the presentations in this volume will be doctors, especially if they are keen to find direct correlations between Western medical knowledge and the tenets of Tibetan medicine. The classification of diseases, their description, the nature of their causes, the way in which therapies are deployed: all of this is profoundly different from what we are used to in the West. Even if in comparison to the period in which this conference took place, and perhaps also because of it, the situation has changed and a few concepts that were new back then are now becoming widespread.

We were able to transcribe most of the presentations that took place in Venice, but unfortunately the material taped in Arcidosso suffered great damage. Those sessions, aside from dealing in depth with some theoretical aspects, entailed mostly moments of practical application that allowed the participants to witness the doctors' work as it unfolded, and to observe them as they dealt with their patients. Special care was given to the issue of mind as element from which both sickness and health can arise, with specific sessions devoted to teachings on our profound nature, as only knowing our real condition we can cut the root from which suffering originates.

Bringing the content of these video tapes to the written page was not easy and required a great commitment, but we believe a book is still an irreplaceable object, even in an image-dominated world like ours has become. Even thirty years later, I remain convinced this effort was worthwhile: those lessons held in the now distant 1983 have lost nothing of their worth and freshness, and thus this text presents us with a knowledge that is timeless.

Luigi Vitiello
November 2015

Preface

The idea of the human being as integration of body, energy, and mind, and of his or her place in both the environmental microcosm and in the planetary macrocosm is common in Eastern philosophies.

Two of the major Asian cultures contributed to the original core of Tibetan culture, namely, the pragmatic essence of Chinese thought and the imaginative fantasy of the Indian spirit, which in turn contributed to the development of the views about people and the world that have shaped the lives of Tibetans until this very day.

Without rejecting or embracing the schematics of Chinese and Indian thought and cosmic visions, Tibetans have produced an understanding of the human condition as a unique chance to realize, in their daily lives, a totality "perfect since the beginning."

In many parts of the world entire cultural traditions have been eradicated. Tibetan culture remained untouched for centuries, but in the last two decades has faced complete annihilation and is currently in a very difficult and delicate phase, even in regard to the gradual disappearance of older generations and to the missed, or incomplete, education of youth. The risk of losing such an unparalleled socio-cultural heritage is quite real.

It is not always possible to draw from the original sources: Tibetan culture gives us a unique opportunity. It is a true privilege to be able to meet the protagonists of this rare and complete human experience, as well as their ideas, their vision of science, and their life practice.

We have now the chance to receive and preserve a great part of this cultural heritage, starting with perhaps its most complete expression, namely its medicine, and to concretely encounter concepts, principles, and methods of application of both the Tibetan and the Western visions.

Venice is the symbol of an already mythical meeting between East and West. This first Conference of Tibetan Medicine offers the possibility of a real bridge between the complete and mysterious Tibetan tradition and our present in progress.

Barrie Simmons

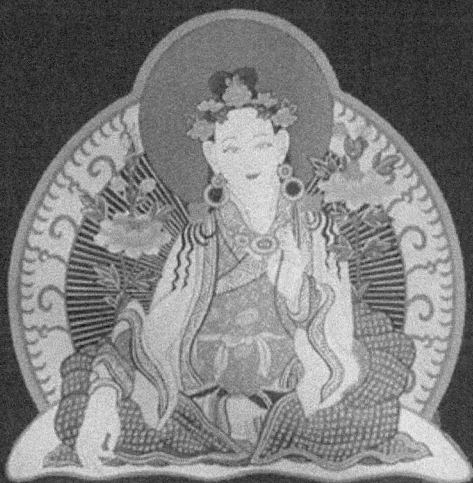

Conference Poster, depicting Yuthog Yönten Gönpo the Elder
(Photo by Luigi Vitiello)

Venice
April 26–30, 1983

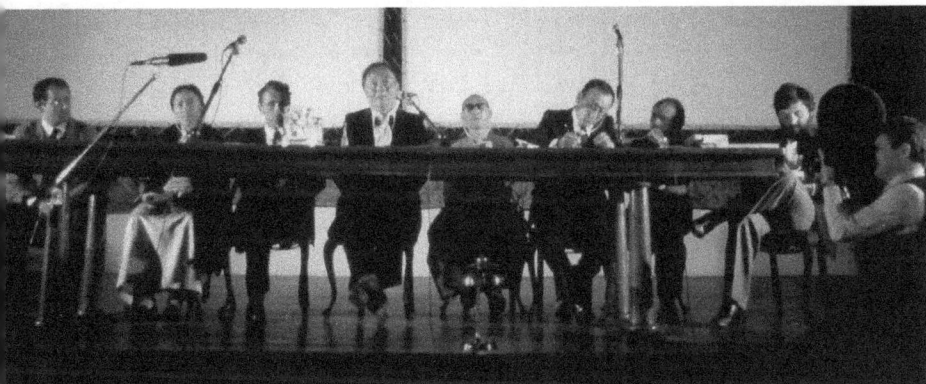

Venice: presenters at the conference (Photo by Ana Maria Humeres)

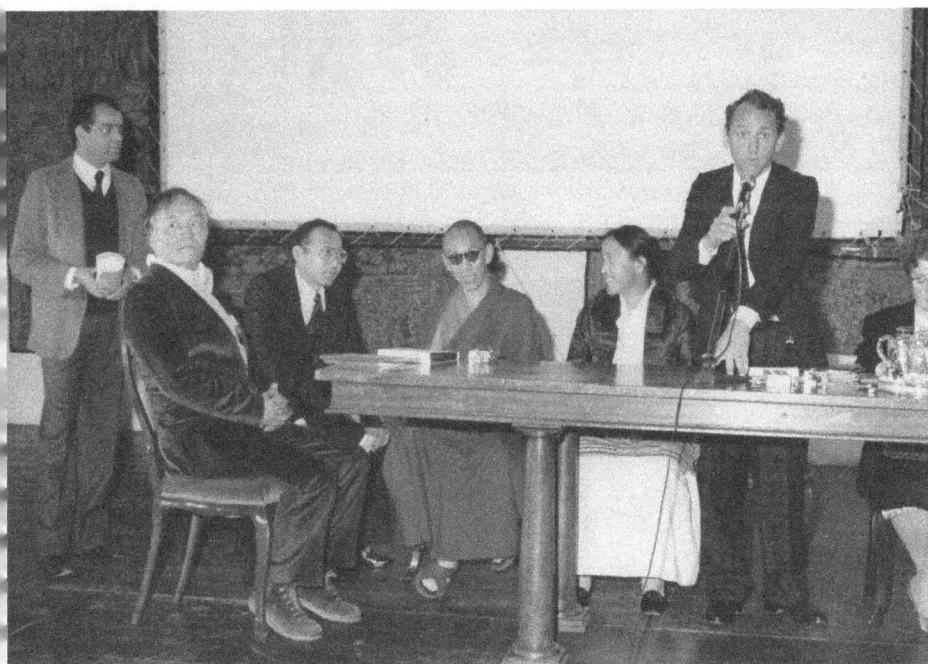

Venice: the inauguration of the conference (Photo by Ana Maria Humeres)

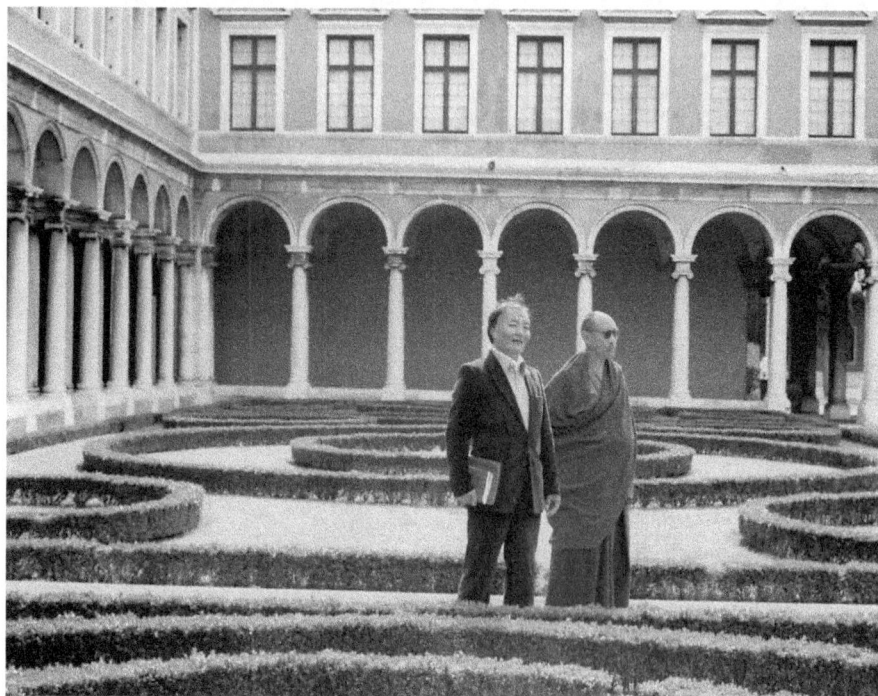

Cloister of the Cini Foundation: Namkhai Norbu and Trogawa Rinpoche
(Photo by Carlos Ramos)

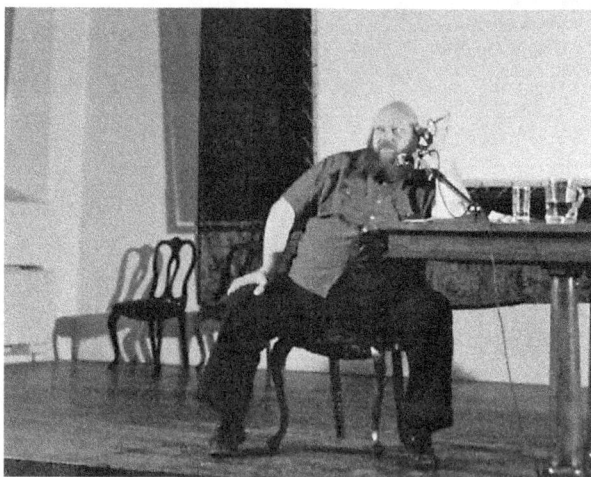

Venice: Barrie Simmons (Photo by Luigi Vitiello)

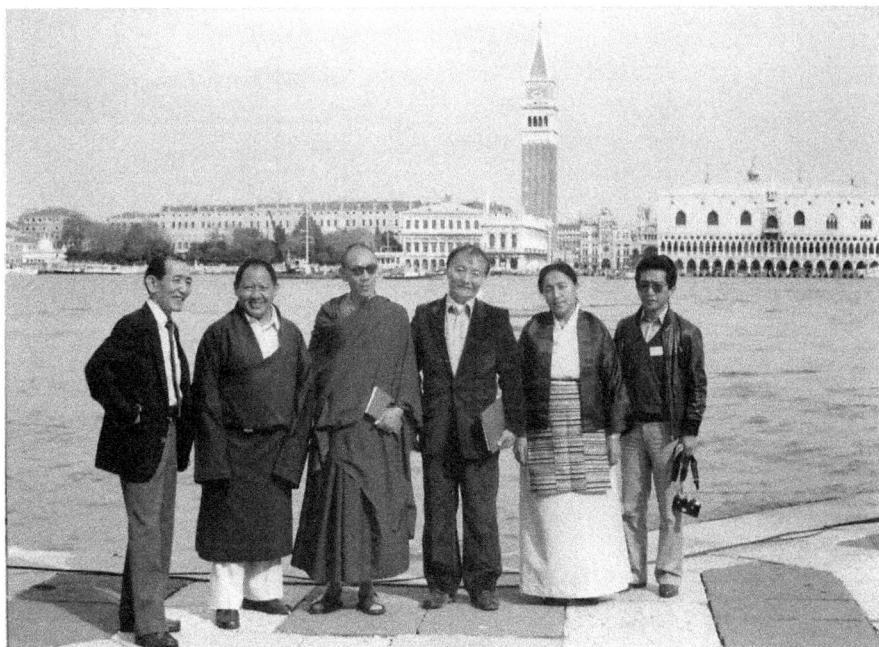

Tibetan presenters at the conference (Photo by Carlos Ramos)

INAUGURATION

Speakers: Doctor Mario Rigo; Doctor Pagnin, Doctor Francesco Guidolin; Marcello Bianchini, JD; Doctor Tsarong Jigme Tsewang; Doctor Ernesto Talentino

Moderator: Architect Paolo Rosa Salva, General Secretary

I would like to invite everyone to take a seat. I now declare this first Conference of Tibetan Medicine in session. At this junction, I believe it is important to call your attention to the cultural climate here in Venice in which this conference is taking place. This year the majority of the cultural events that will take place in the city will be geared towards the engagement with Oriental cultures. Our municipality is organizing a large exhibit in cooperation with the People's Republic of China; the Cini Foundation will organize a high culture course on Eastern themes, and only a few days ago another course on Eastern musical traditions came to a close. I believe it is important to underline that this conference is part of this larger context, and also how our Western culture is discovering an interest in Eastern cultures.

I think that this first meeting on Tibetan medicine has a particular importance because it deals not only with medical questions but also with the question of the preservation of Tibetan culture as a whole. Indeed, from what we hear about the ways in which medicine in Tibet was and is currently practiced, we can infer how tightly this activity is bound to the life style of the people themselves. Therefore, it is relevant not only on the medical level but on the cultural level as well. This is also the rationale for the title of the conference "Man, Medicine, and Society," as it deals with the relationships between people and diagnosis, prognosis, therapy, and social life in general. Before coming quickly to an end, and turning the table to the representatives of local organizations and foundations that have organized the conference, I would like to thank all the different cultural and administrative bodies that have given fundamental contributions to the organization of this event by listing them here in order: the Veneto Regional Administration; the Province of Venice; the Municipality of Venice; the Toscana Regional Administration; the Province of Grosseto; the Municipality of Arcidosso; the Mountain Community of Monte Amiata; and then, in terms of foundations: the Foundation Querini Stampalia; the Foundation Ligabue; the Foundation W. N. Badmajew Stiftung (pro Tibet)-Zurich; the National Research Council [CNR] together with the University of Venice, The University of Siena, and the University of Napoli. The Procuratoria [vestry-board] of San Marco also contributed to the organization of the conference. I thank all of the foundations and the public entities that have contributed in such meaningful manner to the organization of this event, and I now invite the mayor of Venice, Doctor Mario Rigo, to extend the welcome of the city of Venice to the conference participants.

Mario Rigo, Mayor of Venice

I thank Doctor Rosa Salva who opened the conference and who has also diligently contributed to this initiative. There are many institutions that are interested in an issue that has been gathering great interest and great research, as demonstrated by the large number of young people and scholars here at Cini Foundation this morning. It is not common to have to discuss these kind of matters. On the contrary, this, "Man, Medicine, and Society," is the first conference to deal with Tibetan medicine and its cultural and scientific traditions. This is not a common occurrence even for the Mayor of Venice, who has opportunities for international meetings and conferences each week, including with the Middle East and the Far East. You have just heard of the initiatives of the municipality and of the Cini Foundation for next summer's exhibition that will showcase all facets of the formation and the civilization of Ancient China, to be held at Palazzo Ducale, but I will also tell you that this morning at 10, after leaving the organizational meeting for the exhibit, I met a group of young mountain climbers from our region who will attempt to climb the K2 from the Chinese side. I will remind you that it was climbers from Veneto who reached the peak of K2 from the Tibetan side for the first time ever. Nonetheless, today's meeting is still exceptional. And Venice is surely very interested to these questions not only at a superficial level: its historical traditions are so vast and so interconnected with the East that I believe that the proceedings of this conference, in the way they will be documented, will remain in our city, and will enrich on the one hand its knowledge and on the other its archives, already so rich of Eastern sources, so that they will naturally become a subject of research and study for those interested in this issue in the years to come.

What you will discuss today is a theme of extraordinary importance, and I will naturally not speak about it, as I am not competent in this area. There is, however, a passage in the presentation that reads: "It is a privilege to meet the protagonists of this rare and complete human experience, as well as their ideas, their vision of science, and their life practice." I believe this to be truly so. For all the scholars here today I think that it is a true privilege to listen to the protagonists and the heirs of a civilization basically unknown to us, and yet one that has played a great importance in the creation of the Tibetan people's culture. And we believe that civilizations, traditions, have to be preserved with all our strength because they represent our heritage: the heritage of the past, but even more so the heritage that teaches us how to deal with the future. Thank you.

Moderator:

I thank the Mayor and I now invite to speak Mrs. Pagnin, the Alderwoman for Culture of the Province of Venice.

Doctor Pagnin, Alderwoman for Culture, Province of Venice

Doctor Rosa Salva, in his opening speech, has named the cultural institutions and the local groups that with their contribution and patronage
have supported, in part, its organization and promotion. And I believe
that it is important to emphasize, aside from the involvement of cultural institutions, that of local groups, because they demonstrate that
the interest for this initiative, whose purpose the mayor of Venice has
just reminded us, will also provoke, in our view, an interest that will
go well beyond said purpose, and will generate a broader response in
the cultural and scientific fields. Thanks to the information presented
in the press conference we have learned that the aim of this meeting
is basically twofold. The first is to revisit and preserve the heritage of
Tibetan medicine that has remained untouched and has been transmitted over the centuries and that now risks disappearing because the representative of this culture and this medicine are no longer there, and
the new generations have not been able to receive proper training. The
second aim is the aforementioned need to meet the protagonists of this
culture, with their experiences, their practices, and their understanding
of science.

I believe we can also add a third unspoken and implicit purpose for
our gathering, one embedded in our daily tensions and worries, namely
what to do, and how to do it, in order to make our life and medicine
human, so that the progress of Western science, the sophisticated
preparations of our pharmacopeia, the most advanced technologies
of our industry, will not end up dehumanizing their impact on human
beings. The general theme we are drawn to and that brings us together,
a theme that also concerns a little the public administrators, is the
individual, medicine, and society: these three form a triad that need
to remain related, pending the loss of truth and reality existing also in

Western societies. In Eastern culture, based on the little we know and have gleaned from the preparation of the conference, there is a vision of science that sees human beings as an integration of body, energy, and mind; different from our Western understanding which does not include the concept of energy. So now I ask: what have we Westerners lost by ignoring, by not seeing this part? Which bodily and psychic resource have we missed in the healing of human suffering? The wish we have for this gathering is that it will add stimuli and thoughtfulness also to our understanding of science that Eastern people consider more utilitarian than the Eastern one. I recall that Professor Namkhai Norbu said during the press conference: "Western people always ask what something is for; instead, we ask what human beings are, and what is the purpose of the intervention on their bodies and minds." So this is our wish, to have a real exchange between different views of science in a way that may help us solve the common problems that affect our society and our humanity today. Thank you.

Moderator:

I thank Mrs. Pagnin, and I renew our gratitude the Mayor of Venice Mario Rigo, who has now to leave our meeting to carry out his administrative duties. I now invite to speak doctor Francesco Guidolin, the Alderman for Public Health of the Region of Veneto.

Doctor Guidolin, Alderman for Public Health, Region of Veneto

It is my honor to extend, together with my colleague Alderman Conti, the warm welcome of the Region of Veneto to all the illustrious participants of this First International Conference of Tibetan Medicine. Venice, unique in the world for its beauty and famous for its ancient traditions of exchanges with the East and for its culture, is without a doubt the most appropriate venue for this gathering. This congress brings together the most qualified experts and scholars in the world in the field of Tibetan medicine, which is an expression of the global sciences of human beings. Today there is a lot of talk about parallel and alternative medicine. In the face of the scattering of specializations we detect the need to direct medicine towards a global vision of human beings and a more complete knowledge and utilization of the great, and at times mysterious, resources of the human organism. The true medical art is not the one that heals illness but the one that prevents it. I will recall here, especially for the sake of our foreign guests, that in Italy and in Veneto are currently under way health reforms that strongly privilege prevention, as they posit the great source of health in terms of physical, psychic, and social wellbeing of the individual. Medical science is for sure a difficult science, but it is also a fascinating one for those who serve life.

Today I can declare that the Region of Veneto is proud to position itself at the most advanced levels of health care. I can do so because this achievement was made possible by the outstanding scientific and human qualifications of our medical, university, and hospital teams. Our Medical School at the University of Padova, joined last year by the University of Verona, plays an international role and has been one of the first medical schools in the modern world. We are very proud of this, and this is also why, even in the absence of official medicine at this conference, we look with great faith to science without any prejudice, open to all the cultures, like the Tibetan one, that serve mankind. We understand the greatness of Tibetan culture even if, seen from the West, it is shrouded in mystery. But Tibetan culture, together with other Eastern cultures, is a heritage that needs to be defended because it belongs to all humanity.

I would like to conclude my greeting with two very brief reflections. The first is that your first international meeting offers an incredible opportunity for an exchange of ideas and experiences, one that will surely produce positive results for the wellbeing of humanity. He second is that many people will look at this conference of Tibetan medicine as a reference point full of trust and hope. I thank the organizers, especially Doctor Rosa Salva, the members of the Scientific Committee and in particular Professor Carlos Ramos, the drive of this conference. I make the wish that medical science will always triumph, beyond any ideological, cultural, and political boundary, to the service of all human beings. Thank you, have a productive meeting, and enjoy your stay in Venice.

Moderator:

Thank you, Alderman Guidolin, for your kind words, and I now invite to speak Mister Marcello Bianchini, the Mayor of Arcidosso, who will speak also on behalf of the Mountain Community of Monte Amiata.

Marcello Bianchini, Mayor of Arcidosso

One may wonder why the municipality of Arcidosso chose to participate in the First Conference of Tibetan Medicine and to be one of the organizations that have promoted and supported this initiative. The answer is quite simple. First of all, we believe that medicine is culturally ecumenical, and therefore that it does not have territorial, national, and cultural boundaries: medicine is universal. From this basic premise stems the interest of local organizations, such as the Municipality of Arcidosso, which is home to a Dzogchen Community we would like to thank for choosing our town as the stable seat of a permanent cultural center. Consequently, medicine and the initiatives that arise from such a cultural environment are praised by those who feel involved as administrators in a general sense, and that therefore need to be offered knowledge, and the opportunity to gain knowledge to those who have chosen medicine as their way of life and as an opportunity to better their own knowledge for their respective necessities. The other reason that compelled us to participate in this conference is the belief that, beyond the short-term results that will ensue from it, it will draw the attention of the careful, watchful, and interested gaze of the official Italian medical establishment, as well as that of other medical and health-related organizations, which perhaps believe they possess the ultimate cure, the optimal result to cure or heal people as such. This I say because, and I repeat, beyond the short-term results, I believe and we believe that, through dialogue, communication, the opportunities to gather, we create the foundations for a better knowledge of human beings. I do not believe we need to stray far from the theme if we think, for example, how much we need communication between people around the world in this difficult moment, at a time when the threat of nuclear war can and must lead us to reflect on the necessity for an exchange open to all cultures, respectful of each contribution.

I remind you that the conference will hold a second part in Arcidosso on the Second to Seventh of May and of course we invite you to continue to follow the conference with the same degree of attention there as you will do here, in the wonderful city of Venice, because though the conference is split in two parts, they are actually one and the same. Therefore, also Arcidosso is putting at your disposal its limited resources – not as great as those of Venice, of course – so that this important gathering may continue and conclude in the best of ways. I want to thank, as others before me, the organizers of this conference, in particular, but not exclusively, Doctor Carlos Ramos. I am especially indebted to Professor Namkhai Norbu, with whom I have frequent and beneficial exchanges. I thank those who belong to the Dzogchen Community, who have come here in large numbers. I thank the professors who traveled thousands of miles from fascinating faraway countries, and I thank the institutions that together with ours chose to participate in this important initiative, not only in name of the Municipality of Arcidosso but also on behalf of the Mountain Community of Monte Amiata here represented, under a rather exceptional circumstance, by Mister Niso Cini, who has nothing to do with the Cini Foundation. But perhaps this coincidence is a good omen, and I believe it will create the opportunity to ensure that the conference will unfold in the best possible way. I wish everyone a pleasant stay in Venice and I hope also in Arcidosso, and a very productive unfolding of the meetings. Thank you.

Moderator:

I thank Mister Bianchini, the Mayor of Arcidosso. I would like to conclude by stressing the contribution made by the Cini Foundation, represented here by Doctor Talentino, towards the preparation of this conference through all the necessary organizational means, which is typical and exclusive to Venice, also thanks to its branch of studies called "Venice and the Orient." I would also like to thank especially our Tibetan guests because of course a conference on Tibetan medicine would be nothing without their participation, and among them, first of all, I would like to thank Professor Namkhai Norbu who, as you all know, lives in Italy, but thanks to whom we have been able to get in touch with Tibetan doctors living in India and in Tibet. Unfortunately, the doctors traveling from Tibet have not yet arrived. I now invite to speak Professor Jigme Tsarong so that he can share with us his views about this conference.

Tsarong Jigme Tsewang, director of the Men Tsee Khang, the Tibetan Medical Institute of Dharamsala

Secretary General, ladies and gentlemen, on behalf of the Tibetan doctors and of the Tibetan people I would like to thank the public and cultural organizations, the foundations, and especially the citizens of Venice, this wonderful town, for organizing this first historical conference of Tibetan Medicine. Certainly, there is no better site for this event because, as I have learned, Venice is the town of Marco Polo who in the twelfth century built a long-lasting bridge between East and West. Once more you confirm your desire to get to know the Tibetan people, and we return your kind gesture, and I can assure you that, for our part, we will do our best to complete the bridge during this conference, a solid bridge that will benefit humanity. So, again, *grazie*, thank you.

Moderator:

To conclude, I would like to invite to speak Doctor Talentino, our host, to offer greetings on behalf of the Cini Foundation..

Ernesto Talentino, Giorgio Cini Foundation, Venice

Thanks for your invitation: we are very pleased to be included in this set of presentations because they give us the opportunity to say a few words to welcome you all. It goes without saying that the Cini Foundation is extremely pleased to be the site for such a momentous occasion. Professor Ramos knows that we spoke about this initiative something like a year and half ago. All valuable things are a bit difficult, and similarly the gestation process of this conference – as Alderwoman Pagnin and Mister Rosa Salva know – has been a little challenging. And yet, here is the offspring, as it were, of those efforts. And I think that we can be pleased. For sure we will be doubly pleased by the end of the conference, which will then relocate to Arcidosso. I believe that I am entitled to say that the Foundation, even if it has fostered a tradition of encounters with Eastern cultures – for example, we have our own Institute "Venice and the Orient" which deals specifically with languages and literatures – had never dealt with medicine. This is a good opportunity to take notice of the fact that, alas, in life one may get sick, and therefore it is good to include also this aspect in the general conversation about cultures, not only from the medical and scientific angle but also, as everyone has already mentioned, in terms of a global vision of mankind. So the Giorgio Cini Foundation is extremely happy to welcome you and to put at your disposal its structures and my wish is that the conference will not stop its output at the end of the three scheduled days of meetings, but that it will keep on going, and you can already count on the availability of the Foundation for any future continuation. Have a great conference, and have a great stay on the Island of San Giorgio and in Venice. Thank you.

Moderator:

I thank Doctor Talentino for his kind words. I also thank Alderwoman Pagnin and Alderman Guidolin, who will now take their leave because their duties call them elsewhere.

Moderator:

I have the honor of introducing our first speaker, Professor Namkhai Norbu. Professor Norbu was born in eastern Tibet in 1938, and he studied in important monasteries and colleges, where he obtained two university degrees, one in philosophical and literary sciences and one in traditional medicine. He went on to deepen his knowledge in both disciplines by studying on with great teachers of the time, such as Rigdzin Changchub Dorje, his life's inspiration, as well as Khyabjed Kangkar Rinpoche and Khenpo Khyenrab Chökyi Wözer.

In 1959, he went to Sikkim where he taught Tibetan language and literatures to minorities. In 1960, he came to Italy at the invitation of the famous Tibetologist Giuseppe Tucci. Professor Norbu still lives here and teaches Tibetan language and literature at the University of Naples.

In parallel to his duties as teacher of Dzogchen, Professor Norbu is engaged in intense research in the fields of ancient Tibetan history, traditional medicine, life and customs of nomads, and folk traditions, and in so doing he is uncovering and showcasing the historical and scientific heritage of his homeland.

NAMKHAI NORBU
Introduction to Tibetan Medicine

Medicine is one of the most important aspects of Tibetan culture. This culture, like others, has a long history, and the same holds true for its medicine. Therefore, before anything else, I would like to give you an idea of its origins and characteristics. As we know, it is common to think that Tibetan medicine more or less belongs to the Ayurvedic tradition. Indeed, there are principles that hark back to that Indian tradition, but there are also many common elements in ancient Tibetan medicine and the Chinese tradition. On the other hand, it is hard to state that, based on this, Tibetan medicines derives from or has developed from either Chinese or Indian medicine, because to make such a statement one needs a truly global vision of the origins and history of Tibetan medicine.

It is common to date the beginnings of Tibetan history to the spread of Buddhism in the Land of Snows: this is indeed the most widespread idea. But if we study in depth the origins of Tibetan culture we will find something more. For instance, the beginnings of Tibetan medicine originate from a pre-Buddhist system. This means that in Tibet there was an ancient tradition or belief that, in the Western world, would be called shamanism. It predates Buddhism and it is the origin of Tibetan culture, and all aspects of Tibetan culture are based on this tradition. But where did this religion, called Bön, come from? Bön in Tibetan means "to recite," in references to mantras, i.e., magical or secret formulas: this was the principle of that faith or belief.

I have the honor of introducing our first speaker, Professor Namkhai Norbu. Professor Norbu was born in eastern Tibet in 1938, and he studied in important monasteries and colleges, where he obtained two university degrees, one in philosophical and literary sciences and one in traditional medicine. He went on to deepen his knowledge in both disciplines by studying on with great teachers of the time, such as Rigdzin Changchub Dorje, his life's inspiration, as well as Khyabjed Kangkar Rinpoche and Khenpo Khyenrab Chökyi Wözer.

In 1959, he went to Sikkim where he taught Tibetan language and literatures to minorities. In 1960, he came to Italy at the invitation of the famous Tibetologist Giuseppe Tucci. Professor Norbu still lives here and teaches Tibetan language and literature at the University of Naples.

The history of Shang Shung began with the Bön tradition that dates back 3940 years, according to the sources. I have researched this topic extensively, and I will not talk about this now because it is not the main topic of this conference, so I just would like to make you understand that that is the source of the original tradition of Tibetan medicine.

When did the Bön tradition develop? The founder and most important figure of this religion is Shenrab Miwo. According to Bön history, when he was twenty-six years old Shenrab Miwo had a son, Chebu Trishe, who played a fundamental role in the medicine transmitted by Shang Shung, which later became the tradition of Tibetan medicine. How did this happen? Certainly, also through the knowledge of Indian, Buddhist, and Chinese medicine. This is why we need to study and verify the sources.

You know very well the concept of *yin* and *yang*, for instance: today we think that it is a Chinese concept, completely foreign to the Tibetan tradition, but that is not quite accurate. For example, in the ancient Bön tradition, in their rituals, we find the concept of *ye* and *nam*. They are two principles: *ye* is thought to be the origin of the existence of everything and is more or less equivalent to the Chinese *yin*. *Nam* is the manifestation of this origin that can be positive but also negative. This does not mean that *nam* is always negative, but in general we introduce them as positive and negatives forces respectively. The Bön tradition presented them as the origin, truly the original condition and its manifestation. Probably *nam* could be also the Chinese *yang*. I am not saying that this is exactly the case, but when one studies any given culture, when one engages in research, one always finds similarities. Therefore, I think that it is not so important that the Tibetan tradition comes from the Chinese one or the Indian one, or whether it is the Chinese and the Indian traditions that derive form the ancient Tibetan tradition of Shang Shung. Rather, what matters is to understand that we are dealing with a culture and a tradition that truly hark back to ancient times and that holds international value. As a previous presenter explained clearly, Tibetan culture is in the world, and a culture that developed in the world, no matter in which corner of the globe this happened, is a heritage of humankind. Knowing how to use and preserve this heritage is always valuable. Now we have the opportunity to learn and deepen Tibetan medicine through the experience of Tibetan doctors, so in these days we will explain it, and we will endeavor to understand it. Thus, before anything else, it is important to understand that the tradition of Tibetan medicine goes back to an ancient time and that it was already present in the Bön tradition.

Another very important aspect we need to comprehend is that generally, be it in medicine or in the teachings of Tantric Buddhism, we explain what "the individual" means. The individual presents three aspects of existence, as he or she possesses a physical body whose essence is mind, consciousness; but mind and material body are connected by the function of energy. In general, a very commonly used term for energy is "voice." Thus, body, speech, and mind.

Sometimes people do not understand why we say "voice" instead of energy, but for instance in Tantrism it is important to understand the relationship between energy and voice. We are used to seeing material things, and we know an object if it is visible, if we can see it and touch it, and then we have a direct experience of said object, and we find it easy to discover it. But energy is more complex because it is not visible, it is not a material thing, and it is represented through sound, voice. Voice can communicate: when I speak and express an idea in a language we understand, even if what I am saying is not visible and tangible because it is not material, I am able to communicate. This represents the function of energy.

But there is another reason to define energy as "voice." In the individual, voice is connected to breathing. In yoga, in Tantrism, and even in medicine, one of the most important things is breathing. Why? Because breathing is connected to energy, it is a vehicle capable of guiding the function of energy. This is why we define it as "voice," which then comes to mean sound, word, but also our energy. Energy is a fundamental means to communicate and connect the material body to mind.

Generally, especially in the Western world, people have less experience or knowledge of energy, and many do not understand what it means. It is for sure easy to think of electric energy, or to a physical force, for example to the strength of a gigantic person capable of doing many things, but energy should always be understood at this level. Energy moves, but there are many ways to introduce it. For example, in astrology – another important aspect of Tibetan medicine – both in the Chinese and in the ancient Tibetan traditions, we find the Five Elements: namely wood, fire, earth, metal, and water. Wood represents air, because wood refers to the trees that grow and constantly move their leaves in the wind, and this movement is represented by air. Words such as air, water, earth, and so on define the elements directly, but the ancient Bön tradition had a slightly different understanding, and presented them only as force, energy, and stressed their dynamic aspect.

I will give you an example. Usually, as you already know, in the Tibetan tradition we use prayer flags. Many opine that this is a religious belief; others, without understanding why, think that they are beneficial to the individual. On these flags four animals are represented: a tiger, a lion, a dragon, and an eagle or *garuda*. This usage goes back to a very ancient tradition deployed in the Bön rituals, that is, in what today is called shamanism. Why were these images used? Because they represented the force, the energy and the movements of the elements. But why did they not represent energy directly? Why, instead or representing fire as such, did they choose to represent it with an animal? Why, instead of representing air with wood, with trees, did they represent it with a tiger? Because the tiger is a living animal that moves in and inhabits the dimension of the movement of the trees, of the forest. So, this can help you understand why in Bön rituals people used those representations in order to convey the function of elements.

Clearly, the way of seeing of the Bön tradition and the more recent one of the Buddhist tradition are different. We know that nowadays the Bön tradition is heavily influenced by Buddhism. Clearly Bön utilized Buddhist techniques to survive, because when a new culture and a new religion spread in any country problems always arise. This was the case not only in Tibet, but also in the Western world, and we can witness it even today: when Christianity began to spread, many ancient religions and traditions had to change. This happened also in Tibet, and so also the Bönpo [Translator's note: the practitioners of Bön] had to adapt, and this should not surprise us.

So, what do we mean by "the individual"? We mean a being that has body, speech, and mind: these three aspects are present since life begins in the womb. From that moment on Tibetan medicine speaks of *duwa* (*'du ba*), meaning life force, usually translated with the "humors." There are three humors, called in Tibetan *lung*, *tripa*, and *peken*. Usually we translate *lung* with Air, but it does not only mean air, it also means force, energy. *Tripa* is a general term that means Bile, but it may refer both to the bile of the organism and to a specific humor. *Peken* is translated with Phlegm, and it means not only a humor but also, and especially, an active principle with specific characteristics and functions.

For example, as far as the function of the elements is concerned, there are three active elements: fire, air, and water. In Tantrism, in yoga, and various teachings, they are used for purification: fire burns, water cleanses and washes, and the air blows away impurities. These are the three most active elements, and their force corresponds to *lung*, *tripa*, and *peken*, which are not considered an illness, but rather a condition of existence. The human being develops in the womb also thanks to these forces or energies, and, once born, his or her life continues through their balance. When these three energies are balanced, a person is healthy, and if they are out of balance, or in conflict with one another, then sickness develops. As I have already mentioned, these three energies are related to body, speech, and mind, therefore there are no diseases that are exclusively physical, connected to the material body: mind, and especially energy, are involved as well.

In general, in Tibetan medicine there are many analyses of how the various types of diseases arise and develop, but I believe that these topics would be more appropriate for a specific study: if we are only trying to get a general idea, I believe that analyses will make understanding more challenging. In general, medicine is called *men* in Tibetan: this verb means to benefit, and this is really the principle. To benefit whom? Two kinds of individuals: those who are in their own condition, as is, without disturbance, so that they continue to live a healthy life; and those who are in a troubled and problematic condition, and in this latter situation one intervenes depending on the illness. As it is the case with the aspects of our existence, even with diseases we have the three aspects of body, speech, and mind, and there are no diseases that are only about the body. Thus, for the Tibetan doctor the sick person usually cannot be just an object to examine and to whom to prescribe some medicine; one needs to understand the three existences of the sick individual. There are various therapies for this: some work principally on the function of energy, others mainly at the physical level. People usually have a hard time understanding this and they think that the rituals used in the ancient traditions and religions, such as the Buddhist or the Bönpo ones, are prayers in which the faithful believe to gain benefit. But these rituals are not limited to that, they have their own principle based on the knowledge of the function of energy and that can be defined also as science, namely, the science of the knowledge of energy.

In medicine, we talk a lot about a series of illnesses called *dön* (*gdon*), which is usually translated as "disturbance provoked by evil spirits:" many define it this way. This works for those who believe in spirits, but those who do not believe it is not important. This, however, is a principle, a concept connected to energy. In the ancient Bön tradition an individual possesses one positive and one negative force:

when they are balanced, the person is healthy; when they are not, the person gets sick. How can one discover and understand this fact? An individual's balance or lack thereof depends on their circumstances and lifestyle. In medicine, we say that in order to cure an illness, diet, behavior, medicines, and external therapies are fundamental; the first two factors, if they are wrong, become the main cause of sickness. Why are diet and behavior so important? Because they relate to the positive or negative sides of an individual and contribute to create or to disrupt their balance. Therefore, especially in the ancient Bön tradition people studied and acquired a profound experience of the knowledge of this protective force that prevents illness, and they were also able to work with it through rituals. For instance, if the positive side of a person is weak, maybe the person does not get sick, but is in any case very passive and subject to receive negative energies because their force – positive and negative – is related to that of the outside world. Since people live in the dualistic mindset of subject and object there will always be a force that belongs to them and one that belongs to the external world. The force located in the external world is the circumstance of the dimension in which any given individual lives. Then, if the individual's positive force is weak, this person will receive negative energies and things will start to worsen.

In general, we speak of good and bad luck, or of a good or bad time. We do not need to believe in anything in particular to see this, it happens to everybody. We know through our experience that sometimes things go very well, and others they do not, even if we have done everything perfectly. And it is not just one thing that does not go well, everything goes badly and we do not understand why. In medicine, and especially in the ancient Bön tradition, we know that when things go bad we need to reinforce the energies of the individual. There are various ways to achieve this, as well as certain Bön rituals. Of course, rituals seem strange to doctors, but it is important to understand that they have their own principle, and that if they work they have a value – even if we call them magic or shamanism. If the remedy we apply does not work, it has no value, even if we think it is great. Sick people want to be well and get better; they do not care if the cure is magic, a religious ritual, or medicine coming from either Western or Eastern traditions: none of this matters, they just want to get better. Then we need to save them at all costs: doctors need to have this principle and this knowledge.

I recall that a few years ago I attended a conference to speak about Tibetan medicine and that I spoke about the function of mantra to answer a question. Many doctors find the use of mantras strange. It is true, it is strange: in part because a mantra is considered a secret formula. And why should a secret word have a function? It is not easy to explain. It is not easy for Western doctors to understand and accept this because they are used to studying and applying things in a scientific fashion. For them the use of mantra is only a superstitious belief and therefore also the medicine that uses them seems only a belief, a sort of religion. But this is not the case, because words represent our energy, and if they are in written form they have a shape that represents sound, and sound represents our energy. Thus, there are connections. The people who know how to work with this energy find precise answers and are satisfied because they are able to satisfy their desires. For this reason, in Tibetan medicine we use many means, such as medicines and external therapies, but also mantra and meditation because the principle of disease is connected to body, speech, and mind, to all three, and not only to the body. In particular there are many diseases that come from provocations and energy disorders, and from this perspective a fundamental aspect is mind.

We know how many people nowadays suffer from mental disorders! These diseases cannot be healed with medicines alone, everybody knows this. And leaving mind aside, we see this with something as simple as insomnia. Many people suffer from this problem, they cannot sleep at night and so they take sleeping pills. And by taking them every day for months on end they become more nervous and the problem becomes more serious. Why? Because medicines are a material remedy, they work mostly at the physical level, and their capacity to connect and activate energy is minimal. A material thing capable of perfectly activating the energy of an individual does not exist.

If understanding the aspect of energy is hard, understanding mind is even harder. If, for instance, one does not have special clarity, it is hard to understand what the person in front of us is thinking. And why should this be? Because mind is very complicated since it does not have shape, color, or the limits of material things and it is not even like energy. Energy has its own vibration, sometimes there is a way to communicate with sound, but it is not like that for mind. This is why meditation becomes very important. Many people think that meditation has nothing to do with medicine, which usually utilizes concrete and material means. In Tibetan medicine, on the other hand, it is essential to first of all understand what a person is. An individual has body, speech, and mind: these three aspects of existence form a person. When the body, speech, and mind are in their perfect dimension, in their natural condition, one is healthy; when they are not and they are disturbed, then one falls sick.

What must we do when we are sick? We need to find out whether the disease is more related to body, mind, or energy. Afterwards the doctor works on the basis of what is necessary.

In Tibetan medicine, we say that there are 404 diseases (but this is just a synthesis, it does not mean at all that there are only these), divided in 4 groups of 101 each. This division is meaningful and allows us to understand many things.

One group is that of karmic illnesses. In the Buddhist teachings karma is discussed a lot, but it is almost a novelty in the Western world. Karma means action: when you do something, there is a consequence. For instance, in movies there are characters that do bad things and then end up badly. Why? Because evil engenders evil. This is an example of karma. In the Eastern world, most people believe in previous lives; if there are previous lives, there are also consequences to the actions committed in those lives, and if these actions were really negative, there will be consequences in this lifetime, a payback that can manifest in the so-called karmic illnesses.

Many believe that these illnesses are not easy to cure. This is true, but one cannot say that it is impossible: it is just that they cannot be cured with medicine alone. Indeed, if karma is what we are dealing with, one needs to understand of which karma the disease is a consequence. When one understands this, the Buddhist teaching explains that there is a way to purify karma. If one has accumulated negative karma it is possible to purify it, to transform it, or to at least block it, if the individual is aware of it. What does this mean? In Buddhism, karma does not indicate something definitive. When something happens people say: "What can I do? It is my karma!" At times, they call on karma for convenience's sake and they resign themselves to bear it. But this is not how karma works; it is related to our present life, and in our present life we live in a relative condition where there are many conditions related to the ripening of karma.

Let us take the example of the seed of a fruit or of a flower. The seed has the capacity to make a certain flower grow. From the seed of a dahlia a dahlia flower will grow, not another flower or a bean. This is the karmic cause that holds within it a force that can really produce what it is. But the seed alone cannot produce anything: if you keep it in a box, it can sit there for years on end, but it will never grow into a flower. To become a flower it needs soil, water, light, or all circumstances. We usually call these circumstances secondary causes. People live in secondary causes, and if they are aware of them they are also aware of their own karma. Karma matures based on circumstances, and if I know in which circumstances a certain karma can mature I can block it, just like a seed will not grow into a flower if I take away soil or water. Therefore, there are 101 diseases we call karmic, but it is not certain that we cannot overcome them. People do not stop hoping until the very end and always try to do their best.

The second category deals with the 101 illnesses caused by *dön*. *Dön* means not so much evil spirits but negative provocations. Both the *Bön* religion and Buddhism believe that there are many powerful beings that control external energies. As we said earlier, if our positive side is weak we can easily receive negative provocations and illnesses. For instance, we have the deities' *dön,* the nagas' *dön*, the spirits' *dön*, and so on. What does this mean? It does not simply mean that these beings disturb us. In Tibetan "to disturb" translates to *nöpa* (*gnod pa*), and it refers to a different idea. Instead *dön* means that *I* have a part in me open to receive the provocation and then I receive it, and it does not necessarily come from evil spirits, deities, or from other beings: it can come directly from any external energy. This category of illnesses is connected with energy and cannot be cured only with medicine, which becomes secondary in these circumstances: the main cure consists in working on the energy level. Utilizing the force of mantra and rituals is very important to study which provocations we are dealing with and how to address it. So, we should not limit ourselves, it is necessary also to take these matters in consideration.

Another category of 101 illnesses is that of accidental illnesses. They are sudden traumas (for instance a wound or a head bump), and even without using medicine one does not die and can heal. These are occasional illnesses connected to the physical body in particular.

Lastly, the remaining 101 illnesses are called illnesses of life and are tied to the physical body, to the function of energy, and also to mind. Doctors use principally medicines and various external therapies in order to cure them, but it is also important to examine the behavior and the diet of the individual.

These are the basic 404 illnesses discussed in Tibetan medicine. This already gives a precise idea of the fact that in Tibetan medicine we examine the individual in a global fashion.

People often ask me about the relationship between medicine and the Buddhist teachings or astrology. Many things are connected to astrology because astrology is a useful science to understand and deal with the circumstance in which a particular individual ends up.

The same holds true for Yantra Yoga: we know that it includes breathing exercises and movements; there is physical exercise, but there is also meditation; there is a whole series of practices that pertain to the aspects of body, speech, and mind. So it is very useful to stay healthy. Medicine must first of all be used to stay healthy and secondly to solve problems when they manifest.

Tibetan medicine in particular is connected to the Tantric tradition. Perhaps many do not really know what Tantrism is. In the Western world, sometimes it is badly understood, and many think that it is some sort of science of love, but it is not only this. True Tantrism exists especially in Tibetan Buddhism but also in Hinduism. What does Tantra mean? It means "continuity": it is the continuation of the natural state of mind and of its qualifications to manifest energy. It is a condition of the individual, namely the existence of body, speech, and mind that continues without interruption. This knowledge, this condition, is called Tantra. In Tantrism, the fundamental means applied and explained is energy, how the energy of the individual manifests, and how one needs to apply it.

Even in the teachings realization happens through the knowledge of energy and of the means to utilize it; therefore Tantrism has a lot to do with Tibetan medicine. Maybe you know that the fundamental texts of Tibetan medicine are *The Four Tantras*. There are different opinions in this regard: some traditions hold that they were translated into Tibetan from Sanskrit originals, and that therefore they came from India; others posit that they are a sort of summary, of synopsis, of all the medical traditions. But in the end this does not change much; it is not important to judge to see which is the truth. What matters is to understand the meaning of this kind of medicine.

Thus, Tibetan medicine appropriated many tools from Tantrism, especially as far as the function of energy is concerned, but it also absorbed many themes from Buddhism and the Vinaya (the discipline that regulates the life and behavior of monks) as well. In the Vinaya, Buddha often explained subjects related to medicine that later were included in Tibetan medicine, which is then something global and complete that includes elements derived from Tantrism, Sutra Buddhism, Bön, and surely also Chinese and Ayurvedic ideas. People talk a lot about history, so it is not necessary to go into depth about it here.

In conclusion, you are all here not simply out of curiosity or to while away your time. Many of you have come from far away, for example, from the United States, and you are here because of a genuine interest in Tibetan medicine: I am very thankful for this to each and every one of you. I hope that in these days, thanks to the experience of our illustrious guests present here and to their collaboration, you will be able to first of all get a clearer idea of Tibetan medicine. Some people believe that Eastern medicine, especially the Tibetan one, and Western medicine are in conflict, and that the former is positive, the latter negative. But this is not a correct vision: it is better to understand that they can enrich one another. Western medicine is for sure very developed, especially as far as science and technology are concerned, while the Tibetan one is still primitive in this regard. But thanks to Tibetan medicine and teachings like Buddhism and Tantrism, we can have a connection to teachers who, for centuries, have deepened their knowledge of the function of energy, the mind-energy relationship, and most importantly, of the importance of the role that this relationship has for the well-being of the physical body, not only through science but also through the development of their clarity and of meditation.

I hope that you will be able to understand everything very well and that this conference will be truly important, that it will be a new experience that will benefit many beings in the future, just like it is implied in the Tibetan word *men*, medicine, which means "benefit."

Moderator:

It is almost superfluous to thank Professor Norbu, as I believe your applause already expresses gratitude for the clarity in which he has conducted this introduction to Tibetan medicine.
Ritengo quasi superfluo ringraziare il professor Norbu, penso che l'applauso sia significativo per la chiarezza con cui ha svolto questa introduzione alla medicina tibetana.

Venice, April 26, 1983
Afternoon (first session)

Moderator:

Tsarong Jigme was born in Tibet, and he is a writer specializing in Tibetan medicine. He was the director of the Men Tsee Khang, Tibetan Medical Institute of Dharamsala, from 1975 to 1980. Doctor Jigme, if you please.

TSARONG JIGME
The Fundamental Principles of Tibetan Medicine

Good afternoon, everyone. First of all, I would like to say a few words about the history of Tibetan medicine. I will do my best to try and be as simple as possible in my explanation. Secondly, I will talk about the fundamental principles that are at the base of this system of medicine, and, always in regards to theory, I will talk about the three vital processes from a spiritual or mental point of view. Then I will talk about the five proto elements that are at the basis of matter, as well as of its vitality, since we are dealing with a holistic vision that runs counter to the modern mechanistic way of understanding life. Thirdly, I will deal with practice, treatments, and ways to heal patients such as diet, life style, and other forms of external therapy.

To begin with it is important to explain what Tibetan medicine is and what its actual origins are. This morning we heard Professor Norbu speak about the origins. In the manuscripts we have at our disposal we find mention of massage, a rudimental form of pulse diagnosis, and also some use of medicinal oils, but the medicine actually practiced is mostly based on the Buddhist system of medicine, and this is why we speak of Tibetan medicine. It is true that this system developed in Tibet, but we have to go back to its origins. It is commonly believed that it originated in India. Because medicine is Dharma, one cannot separate the two, and the original Dharma teachings come from Buddha. I think that in order to understand Tibetan medicine one should understand all so called "Buddhist" religions. I would prefer to call them lifestyles and not necessarily religions, since we are dealing here with a way of life whose fundamental idea is that there is an imperfection in the world; that all of us, in some way and at various moments in our lives have to deal with pain and suffering; that our life is not permanent, and it changes constantly. Our loved ones will leave us, and our life, if we are lucky, will last one hundred years and not much longer, and therefore our life is nothing but a fragment in the cycle of time.

Why are we living in time? Why do we all suffer? Because we are all afflicted by passions. Therefore, technically, we are all sick because we have not realized liberation. This is what Buddha tried to do, namely to find a way to reach liberation. Thus, all the theory of Tibetan medicine is centered on the idea of suffering. And what is suffering? The technical Tibetan term is *marigpa* or *dagzin*, the attachment to oneself, to the ego each of us has. And this ego, that some translate as ignorance, confusion, or disorientation, is the source of insatiability, desire, dissatisfaction with everything, of ambition, greed, and the quest for power. This we call *döchag* or attachment: we all have it, and from attachment also *shedang* is born, that is, the capacity human beings have to hate one another, or aggression. These are the imperfections. So, the general idea is that we possess both positive and negative aspects: good and evil are within each of us, and our objective is to develop the positive aspects and achieve liberation this way.

So, in relation to the spiritual aspect, these are the causes of the original humors, *lung*, *tripa*, and *peken*. Therefore, human beings suffer from a disturbance and call them illness [Fig. 1].

Now, we have the spiritual or mental factor and one material or physical. From the mental side of things, we have the three poisons, *döchag*, *shedang*, and *timug*, namely, attachment, hatred or aversion, and confusion or ignorance. In correspondence to the three poisons we find the three vital processes, not the three humors; this is a big mistake we all make. The idea of humors comes from the Greeks, from the original idea of Aristoteles, later picked up by the Arabs, and developed into the Unani system.[1] From here stems the concept of humor: individuals may be phlegmatic, melancholic, or sanguine. The idea of the four humors spread, and the Ayurveda began to use the same idea and to speak about

---

1   Unani is a form of alternative medicine based on the idea that the human body contains four humors (blood, phlegm, yellow bile, and black bile), and that the cause of illness is the lack of balance among these four humors.

3 Vital processes		5 Proto-elements	3 Vital processes
Lung	← 1. ATTACHMENT	EARTH	$\Big>$ Peken
Tripa	← 2. ANGER	WATER	
Peken	← 3. IGNORANCE	FIRE	→ Tripa
		AIR	→ Lung
		SPACE	→ Lung

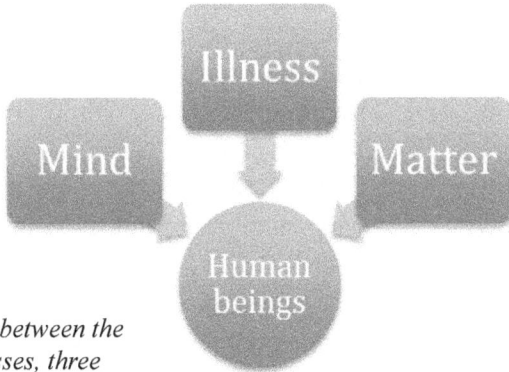

Figure 1
The relationship between the three vital processes, three emotions and five proto-elements

bile, phlegm, and air. Some Tibetan translators also fell in the same trap and began to use the same term, but the three vital processes have nothing to do with humors. This is how the confusion began: we are dealing simply with *lung*, *tripa*, and *peken*, I do not believe that they can be translated.

So, from attachment we get *lung*, from hatred *tripa*, and from ignorance *peken*. These are the three vital processes within us. I do not believe that *peken* is a Tibetan word, and I think that it is corruption of the original Arabic term *bal-gam*, which means earth and water. I have allowed myself to diverge from the historical sources we were talking about, and moved to this theory. In any case what I explained is related to the point of view of mind.

Now, from the point of view of matter, we have the five proto-elements: Earth, Water, Fire, Air, and Space or *namkha* – to simply call them the five elements could create confusion with the elements that we know. How do the three vital processes relate to matter? Earth and Water generate *peken*, Fire *tripa*, and Air *lung*, and so we have the three processes once more. This is the theoretical foundation of Tibetan medicine.

This morning we spoke a lot of energy. Of course, we have mental energy and elemental energy. Now, to apply all of this to a concept familiar to us, let us consider the foundation of matter, and take, for instance, a hydrogen atom. We have one positive and one negative, namely the electron (-) rotating around the nucleus (+). The nucleus is a compounded element, but it is solid, made of earth and water combined. Now, the electron does not move by itself, a force must be present for movement to occur. And what is this force? It is movement, energy, in other words, Air. When movement is present, there is always a release of heat, and so we have Fire. And all of this would not exist without Space, which is a necessary factor. This is the basis of matter.

The biggest problem of today's modern orthodox medicine is that it acknowledges only one part, matter, and not the other, mind, which medicine is starting to engage only now. It sees human beings as only matter that can be explained with physical and chemical laws. It is interesting, however, that at times, when one goes to a doctor because one is unwell, he or she will say that everything is fine, after conducting a normal check-up, with X-rays, lung auscultation, blood pressure check, and blood and feces analyses. But the patient knows that something is not right. That means that on the mental end of things you have a lung disorder. *Lung* illnesses can be treated with medicine, and naturally, also through spiritual teachings. This is a fundamental point.

Furthermore, pharmacopeia is based on matter, not on spirit. Tibetan medicine acknowledges mind, but in practical terms it deals more with matter. As far as medicaments are concerned, the four elements have specific characteristics: they have *nupa*, which means the dynamic principle or action from which the six flavors derive. I will talk about this later, when I speak about pharmacopeia. Mind and matter are the basis: the two pillars of Tibetan medicine.

Before delving into this, I would like to add something I left out about history. Among the four great traditions of humankind there are three great civilizations, namely the Mediterranean, the Indian, and the Chinese one. The fourth one, the civilization of Central Asia, is a bit later. Each of these civilizations developed a medical system. In the Mediterranean civilization, as I have already explained, there was the great Greek medical tradition; this was later absorbed by the Arabic-Persian culture and is known as the Unani system. In India or in Southern Asia, we have the Indian system of Ayurveda, the science of life. *Ayur* means life, *veda* means science. And then we have Chinese medicine. Nobody speaks of Tibetan or Buddhist medicine. Now it is simply called Tibetan medicine because we Tibetans, after introducing it from India, have gone on to develop, synthesize, and practice it, so much so that today it is widely known as the system of Tibetan medicine. But technically it all goes back to the Buddhist idea, it is the original system of Buddhist medicine. Nowadays, since Tibet has been colonized, the Chinese state that it is Chinese medicine. And since we, Tibetans, are refugees in India, the Indians say that it is Ayurvedic medicine. Then there are small nations that claim it as their own, like for example Ladakh ("This is Ladakhi medicine, amchi medicine."). The Bhutanese say that it is Bhutanese medicine, while the Mongols practice it like Mongolian medicine. At any rate, no matter what it is, the fact remains that in Tibet we have preserved and developed it, and not like a dogmatic teaching, but as an eclectic system of knowledge. The basic theoretical elements are the same: the theoretical foundation has remained more or less the same of the period of the Second Yuthog Yönten Gönpo, who lived in the twelfth century, because it is founded on the *Gyüzhi*, *The Four Tantras*, but the greatest development is to be found in the pharmacopeia. If you compare these three or four civilizations, also the civilization of Central Asia developed a medical system, but today this system is no longer present in the various conferences on traditional medicine promoted by the World Health Organization. In the last eight years I have tried to spread the idea that Tibetan medicine is important, but it is not recognized yet. The reason is always political. Since Tibet has been colonized by the People's Republic of China, its medicine has become Chinese medicine: this is the problem we have, this is our reality.

Now, why are the four great medical traditions so great? Because they have an academic basis: we have manuscripts, scriptures, and they are practiced. Chinese medicine, Indian Ayurveda, Unani, they all have their own textual sources. But why is the Tibetan medical system so important? I think that we must find the answer not so much in the idea that

Tibetans are more intelligent or something like that, as the answer lies in the geographical isolation of Tibet. Here we had a medical system whose philosophical foundations lay in Buddhism and that came together with a native system that in turn had absorbed ideas from Mongolia, China, and also Persia, as we can gather from the Arabic word *bal-gam*. At the time of Songtsen Gampo, in the sixth century CE, we find mention of the arrival of Galenos, a Persian doctor – not the famous Galenos, just someone else by the same name – for the gathering of doctors. At that time, from the sixth to the eighth century CE, Tibetan kings were very interested in medicine. And even earlier during Ashoka's reign in India the medical system had developed, and it was one completely compatible with Buddhist philosophy because it was entirely based on the compassion towards the patient. Ashoka lived around the third century CE and is said to have been the first to build hospitals. Afterwards there was Kanishka, a first century CE Indian king, whose famous doctor was Charaka. They were all Buddhists. Later the famous Tibetan kings Songtsen Gampo and Trisong Deutsen were great patrons of Tibetan medicine, and thanks to them the medical system flourished.

Now we are holding the first international congress of Tibetan medicine, but if we look at history, there were also such gatherings between the sixth to the eighth century CE: many famous doctors were invited to Tibet from India, China, Mongolia, and they brought along the translation of a compendium of the best works that the kings had commissioned. The Tibetan doctors examined these sources, and introduced them into their system and they adapted them to the local medicine and philosophy so that they developed in this way. Perhaps those were the first international congresses of medicine ever recorded in history.

Nowadays Tibetan medicine is becoming very important because it is a complete medical practice and an uninterrupted system due to Tibet's geographical isolation as well. Unani and Ayurveda once had good traditions, but then their respective countries were occupied and fanatic invaders looted their famous libraries, and thus today, in comparison, those systems no longer have truly original texts, whereas materials abound in the Tibetan medical system. Our medicine included more than one thousand manuscripts, and even with the Chinese invasion of Tibet, the looting of monasteries and the destruction of manuscripts, I believe that it is very important that there are still two or three hundred medical texts left.

Another reason why Tibetan medicine is important is that its uninterrupted practice is related to our system or our tradition of Tantra: its continuity is due to the transmission of knowledge from teacher to student so that, even nowadays, the official Tibetan doctors can date back their lineage to the times of Buddha. I believe that this is a very important aspect of Tibetan medicine.

I would like to say something more about history. There is a theory that the *Gyüzhi* were translated into Tibetan from another language. But they cannot be a translation from Sanskrit because there is no original Sanskrit manuscript. If we probe the question more in depth, the diet and the plants described in the *Gyüzhi* are mostly native to Tibet, aside from the spices that are of course grown in India. For instance, yak, *tsampa*, *chang,* and so on do not exist in India, and yet they are still mentioned in the *Gyüzhi*. Then there is the Chinese influence on the pulse that in my view deals mostly with the astrological aspect, the influence of the *nagtsi* (*nag rtsi*), one of the two astrological systems that we have absorbed and utilize a lot for the pulse. In the chapter about the pulse we have Chinese words: they are not Tibetan words, but we find them in the *Gyüzhi*, and therefore these cannot originally have been in an Indian text. At any rate I am only speculating, this is a theory of mine.

I believe that the Buddhist teachings already included the fundamental ideas for medicine, and the *Gyüzhi* were later translated by Vairochana at the time of Trisong Deutsen, in the eighth century.[2] They were then given to Yuthog Yönten Gönpo, the most famous Tibetan doctor – that many believe was the second Medicine Buddha – who transmitted his knowledge to his son, and his son in turn to his son, and so on and so forth, until the Second Yuthog Yönten Gönpo, who edited what his ancestor had done. Therefore, we can comfortably say that the *Gyüzhi* that we

---

2   More information on this subject can be found in the lecture of Doctor Trogawa Rinpoche.

have today date back to the Second Yuthog Yönten Gönpo and that the entirety of Tibetan medicine is founded on these sources.

Let us move on now to the treatments. What happens when someone gets sick? We have now to introduce the concept of "balance." We believe that the above-mentioned energies can easily be altered by the excess of one or the lack of another, and therefore the concept of balance is always present. We think that the body exists in a very delicate state of balance. These energies are known as *gyu*, primordial causes. Therefore, we can apply this theory to anything. To obtain a fruit we must have an original cause, the cause that brings about the effect. But the original cause will not bring fruit unless other factors come into play. For example, in the three vital processes we have *lung, tripa*, and *peken*; all of us have them. We can be by nature a *lung* or *tripa* or *peken* person, or we could be *lung-tripa*, or *lung-peken*, or we can have all three of them together. Generally, we say that a *lung* individual is by nature of dark complexion, very nervous, and small boned. Other individuals are very accommodating, perhaps a bit lazy, and remain calm even if you harass them: their nature is *peken*. And then there are the combinations [of these three humors]. Everyone has the three humors, it is a universal condition. So there must be a triggering factor without which there will be no illness.

What are the factors that can cause the arising of a disease? Our vital processes can become unbalanced as a result of food or from an inappropriate diet, from an inappropriate behavior or life-style, and also from *dön* or negative factor we discussed this morning. Some people translate *dön* as evil spirits or demons, but it really means negative factor, damaging force. It cannot be explained; it just happens. These are the triggering factors, and it is easy to understand them, because if you eat inappropriate food you get sick – you get diarrhea or a stomach-ache. If your lifestyle is very frenzied and you are under stress, you will feel stress, anxiety, depression. There has to be the contribution of these factors to have the outcome. Our theory is that if the body is balanced, in a state of homeostasis, the body will be able to repel any kind of bacteria or virus: it has the immune system, a defense mechanism able to destroy them. You can verify this by exposing some people to a virus or bacterium: some will get sick, others won't. If there is a flu outbreak, some will not get sick because their immune system is strong. And so we believe that regardless of the nature of the pathogen, if the ground is fertile it will grow, if it is not, the pathogen will not thrive.

Then we have the medicines made from ingredients of various kinds: minerals we call *do* or *sa*; vegetal ones like resins, shrubs, and plants; animal extracts; precious materials called *rinpoche*: for instance, gold, rubies, and turquoise belong to this category. We use minerals like serpentine, realgar, mica, and so on, and specific minerals extracted from the soil. We utilize plants like pomegranate, sandalwood, and pine. Then we use *tsi* which include resins but also bear bile and deer musk. Then we have shrubs like licorice, and of course herbs like saffron, delphinium, and so on. As for the animal extracts we deploy the hearts of various animals, fish liver, fish bones, and so on. These are the coarse basic materials normally used to prepare various remedies. Usually people are familiar only with pills, and they believe that round pills are all that we use in Tibetan medicine, but this is not the case: we also have decoctions, ointments, medicinal oils, soups, and medical wines, and the precious pills *rinchen rilbu*. We make all these with our ingredients.

All of our pharmacopeia is based, as I explained earlier, on the five proto-elements, each of which has specific properties and actions. Then we also use the six flavors. Speaking of which, I would like to say that also in Ayurveda we find the six flavors, as well as the three vital processes (*lung, tripa, peken*), and the seven constituents of the body I have not mentioned. Some aspects are similar, so some people say that Tibetan medicine is Ayurveda, but if we examine things carefully, also the flavors and their related applications are different. We have the sweet, salty, spicy, acid, sour, and bitter flavors, and therefore they are different [from the ones in Ayurveda, which are sweet, sour, salty, pungent, bitter, and astringent].

Tibetan medicine also has eight branches, the eight classifications, and this is surprising because the classification system in medicine began only in the nineteenth century, whereas the *Gyüzhi* dates back to the twelfth century and already includes the eight-branched classification. Ayurveda has eight branches as well, but we differ in some areas. For example, if we look at mind, Ayurveda does not consider it: it does not explain mind. Our idea of mind is based on Buddhist philosophy, on the three poisons, and they do not have this, and what they say is based on the three deities: Brahma, Shiva, and Vishnu. Therefore, their explanations are very different. And, even more to the point, we believe that mind is much superior to matter because all of us – material bodies – will quickly be gone because the wheel of time is nothing but a snap of the fingers. We believe that mind continues and that, through our actions, we are able to develop: it is in the power of each of us to improve and to gain liberation – there is no fatalism. Some of you are perhaps familiar with the wheel of samsaric existence: all those who are in the wheel of life share the condition of suffering, and the aim is to leave samsaric existence. In these points we differ from Ayurveda.

Now I would like to say something about the eight branches of medicine discussed in the text:

1. First, we have *lü*, which is the physical body per se, and encompasses general pathology, anatomy, embryology, pharmacology, and so on. All these aspects are included in *lü*;

2. Pediatrics;

3. Gynecology;

4. *Dön* and negative forces that are also contemplated in Ayurveda;

5. Treatment of wounds;

6. Toxicology. This branch in quite advanced in my view, perhaps because in the past poisoning was quite common: kings were poisoned, conspiracies were quite widespread, and so doctors had to work hard at prevention;

7. Geriatrics, the treatment of old age;

8. Fertility. Some use the terms aphrodisiacs for this branch, but I believe that we are dealing here with the idea of fertility.

These are the eight branches of medicine. Why eight? We opine that it is because they are tightly connected to the eight-fold noble path of Buddhist philosophy.

Together with the medications we have various external therapies such as phlebotomy, bloodletting, moxabustion (different from the Chinese one,

Tsarong Jigme ▪ 65

as at times we use gold tools and rely on different meridians), hot and cold patches, massage, and gold needle therapy, which leads many people to say we have acupuncture in Tibetan medicine, but as far as I know we do not practice it. We only use one point on the top of the head, called *tsangpai buga* or Brahma's door, to apply the golden needle and cause the heat to descend. This is also the spot from which consciousness exits the body at death. A Tibetan about to die can have a lama who conducts the so-called *phowa* to make the dying person's consciousness leave the body. For example, in Tibet, in the Drikung Kagyud tradition, many lamas specialize in *phowa*. I gather that some lamas, such as Ayang Rinpoche and others, do this also in Europe. And when they do it you can see the hole on the top of the head, and therefore you can believe that it is true. Many are skeptical, and when they see the hole produced only by the invocations of the lama they are astounded. Yet it is there, quite visible.

Then we have thermal water therapies.

Tibet has also some form of surgery, but it is not very developed. We practice some cuts, some drilling, but it is underdeveloped; it is not a refined practice like in modern medicine. How come? It is said, without any actual historical proof, that once a queen died as a result of a surgical procedure and that since then the king banned surgery. I do not hold this theory to be true, and rather believe that the truth is that the Buddhist medical system underlines how the body is a very delicate organism, that its balance is delicate, and the idea is to treat this balance with care. This is very important. Surgery is a drastic way to intervene, therefore Tibetan medicine first of all tries to suggest the correct diet and the right lifestyle advice. Then, if it is necessary to take medicine, the doctor will prescribe something very bland, like a concoction, and if this does not work, as a last resort we use pills. Therefore, a blend approach to medicine is very important.

Besides, we use only natural medicines without anything synthetic. And we do not allow the use of one plant only either because the effect can be very strong. If it is necessary, then it is ok, but one must avoid this approach as much as possible. So for us it is surprising to witness how modern medicine works; namely that you get the most active ingredient from one plant, you attempt to synthesize it, and you administer it to the patient. Hence, once more, there is a difference from the philosophical point of view. For this reason, in Tibetan medicine we have many ingredients and we try to balance medications: if an ingredient is very toxic, we add another to balance the effect of the former.

In general, the majority of Tibetan medicines are made of eight, nine, or ten ingredients. And the most famous Tibetan remedy, *rilnag chenpo,* the great black pill which we are still unable to make, has 116 ingredients. On top of this, it requires mercury – a mercury base specifically purified with a process that I will show you phases of in a slide presentation on the twenty-ninth of April. And, of course, we need equipment and instruments, and so technically we have two hundred ingredients in only one medicine. We are planning to produce it at Dharamsala, at the Tibetan Medical Institute – the official Tibetan medical center of His Holiness the Dalai Lama. They have already produced a couple that I will show you pictures of.

I have left out a very important point that, naturally, the doctors will talk about extensively, and that is how we diagnose patients. I have explained the theory and the historical background, and now I will give you a general approach to Tibetan medicine in a way that everyone can understand it and hopefully appreciate it.

How do you diagnose patients? There are three main methods. The first is visual: we visit the patient and check his or her eyes and tongue. The tongue is a very important element, as it reveals a lot. Urine too is very important: a doctor can understand from it if the patient is more influenced by *lung* or *tripa.* For instance, in the case of a *lung* disorder, if you stir the urine [with a stick] its color will be blue-whitish, big bubbles will form, and its smell will not be so strong as it would be if the ailment is related to *tripa.* If you check the *lung* by looking at the tongue, you will see that [in the case of a *lung* ailment] the tongue will have many small dots on both its sides. Visual examination is very important when dealing with children because technically you cannot examine the pulse of children under ten or twelve years, and Doctor Trogawa Rinpoche will explain this more tomorrow: we check instead the ear veins by placing the child with the sun behind so as to see the veins better.

Last but not least there is the famous pulse diagnosis. A few years ago, I read in one of the major Indian newspapers an article entitled "The Death of Pulse Diagnosis." It dealt with the Indian system, and how they lost this art, which today has almost completely been replaced by the stethoscope. I intended to write to the newspaper to say that pulse diagnosis is still alive and kicking, but I never got around to it. In any case we still practice it; the art of pulse diagnosis exists still nowadays and it is very interesting. Perhaps, at the end of the conference, the people in attendance who have some illness can ask the doctors to diagnose them to satisfy their curiosity. How is it done? I believe that Doctor Trogawa Rinpoche will talk about it. The Tibetan way to check the pulse is different from the Chinese one. Of course, if we get technical, we find certain similarities, but the Chinese have the Triple Burner and The Heart Master – two of the twelve Meridians in Chinese medicine that have no correspondence in our system. So, differences notwithstanding, the Chinese say that our pulse diagnosis is an ancient system of Chinese medicine. At any rate, the chapter on the pulse is only one of the 156 chapters in the *Gyüzhi*, and therefore there is some influence from Chinese medicine, but Tibetan medicine is not Chinese medicine.

Finally, there are the questions that the doctor must ask the patient. Especially in India our doctors are famous for having patients who do not talk to them and just show them their wrists: and this is not good. I believe that our doctors have spoiled them because they immediately check the patient's pulse, and then they diagnose them, and the patient is impressed. But the true diagnostic method according to our tradition includes all of these three methods, and needs to be done accurately, and this means asking the patient questions, looking at him, examining him, examine him and checking the pulse.

I have given you a short and generic introduction to Tibetan medicine, and tomorrow the doctors will deal with the details. Are there any questions?

Questions and Answers

Question: I would like to know if in Tibet there is a tradition related to alchemy, especially in the preparation of medicines.

Answer: In Tibet, we do not use chemical medicines. As I said earlier, everything is based on the five proto-elements from which the six flavors derive. For example, if someone suffers from lack of appetite, it is a disorder related to cold. So to counterbalance it we then administer medicines that have a heating effect, so as to balance cold and heat again; or we administer something light and rough, always to counterbalance the ailment. For something that is fat we administer something absorbent, and this is what our pharmacopeia is based on. We have however specific medicines that contain some potentially toxic minerals that are modified to eliminate their toxicity with a specific process.

Question: Could you specify the difference between mind and what we call the mental? At times, there is a great deal of confusion between these two terms, and especially in Chinese medicine these two terms have a particular meaning. What is your take on it?

Answer: Mind and mental event are a topic I am not really qualified to talk about, you should direct your question to Doctor Trogawa Rinpoche.

Question: Could you explain to us the difference between gold and silver and their qualities in needles? In Chinese medicine the material acupuncture needles are made of is not that important. Thank you.

Answer: Gold is good for long life, for poison, and age defying purposes; it dries fluids, ligaments, and joints. Ama Lobsang can speak more about the qualities of silver.

Question: Do you use only the heated golden needle for application on the head or also the silver one?

Answer: Also the silver one.

Question: You mentioned that the reasons for attachment and hatred depend on nature. What do you think about the causes of interpersonal unconscious processes, such as when a person hurts us not physically but psychically? Why does a person experience more attachment, another more hatred, and a third a mixture of these two factors that are the basis for interpersonal relationships?

Answer: I think that it depends a lot on personality, we react in different ways: some people may feel more hatred than others. But the general idea is that we all have these afflictions or emotions – *nyepa* in Tibetan – that drive us to be reborn in the cycle of transmigration. We all feel them, but they can vary from person to person, because we have *lung* people, and so on; as I have already explained there are seven types of people.

Question: So there is a reaction due to an interpersonal process, and not to nature?

Answer: It is in everyone's nature, perhaps dormant; but we react in different ways. In some cases, one can hit a person and then ask one-self: "Why did I just do that?" So, the idea or lifestyle of the Buddhist tradition is to develop positive aspects. One can also have specific negative forces, something karmic stemming from previous lives, so the idea is to develop positive aspects.

Question: Is it possible to cure cancer by diagnosing someone from a distance, without having one photo of the patient, and to treat him without giving him medicines?

Answer: It has been done. In the pulse diagnosis there is an entire section or chapter on the pulse with thirteen sections. One of these is known as *ngotshar tsadün*, the seven wonderful pulses. It is not something all doctors can do, as it requires a great deal of practice, a certain natural gift that some have and others can learn. For example, we have the case of a father who is not with the doctor because he is far away, so one can take the son's pulse and then, in terms of the organ that pulses, the doctor can at least say whether the father can be healed. As I said, only a very special doctor can do this. Some can also foretell the length of a person's life, meaning that they can predict when a person will die.

Question: But if a person lives, say, 5,000 kilometers away, can a Tibetan doctor diagnose what is wrong with that person, if anything? Even without know that person's name?

Answer: I don't think so. I do not think that the distance is important, be it ten or twenty thousand kilometers, but the doctor needs to have access to a relative, the wife, or the son, so through their pulse the doctor can diagnose the absent patient.

Venice, April 26, 1983
Afternoon (second session)

Moderator:

Trogawa Samphel Rinpoche was born in 1931 in Lhasa where, since his youth, he learned to write and to practice the Dharma. When he was sixteen, he became the student of the famous doctor Nyerongsha Rigdzin Lhundrub Paljor, who had studied with Khenpo Ampa Thubwang, the personal doctor of the Thirteenth Dalai Lama. He studied with Nyerongsha for nine years, learning the Tibetan medical art in all its aspects, and became a practicing doctor at the age of twenty-one in Lhasa and its surroundings. He also taught for three years at the Tibetan School of Medicine and Astrology in Dharamsala, India.

TROGAWA RINPOCHE
History of Tibetan Medicine: Medicine and Dharma

I would like to extend my greetings to everyone here. The culture of Tibet is very ancient, and has undergone various different historical periods, each of which had its unique contribution. Medicine developed from the very beginnings of Tibetan culture. It is true that we find medicine in all of the cultures of the world, and this is due to the fact that beings live in a condition of ignorance, and in this condition they suffer because of a variety of illnesses, so their natural impulse is to try and find a cure. Therefore since antiquity the medicine is one of the main factors in all civilizations, including the Tibetan one. Transmitted in writing in the Tibetan language it is today a codified and organized science, and consists of traditions that originated or developed inside Tibet. Tibet is a country enclosed by majestic peaks that surround it like a necklace of pearls, and the various medical developments that took place within it are included in Tibetan medical science which contains elements characteristic and unique to Tibet, but also some in common with other medical systems.

I would like to speak a bit about this latter aspect, namely about the medical knowledge imported from other countries, beginning with India. In ancient India there were two practical systems to apply medicine: the Brahmin system and the Deva system. A great teacher of medicine in ancient India, Biji Gaje, master in both systems of medicine, had a vision of a deity, and following the deity's instructions went on a trip to Tibet during the reign of Lha Thothori Nyantsan (245–364 CE). Lha Thothori Nyantsan welcomed Biji Gaje with great honors, giving him great presents, including his own daughter as wife, and persuaded him to stay in Tibet for the rest of his life. Biji Gaje remained in Tibet for a long time practicing medicine and greatly benefiting Tibetan people. He had one son, Dungi Thorchog, and since then the history of medicine in Tibet has been strictly connected to that of its rulers.

In the seventh century CE the great king Songtsen Gampo (617–650 CE) ruled the country of Tibet, which was then a very powerful nation equal to China. The king's wife was Chinese, and her name was Kong-jo. Thanks to her influence, many texts of medicine and astrology were translated into Tibetan. Furthermore, in that time, doctors from Nepal, Kashmir, India, Iran, Shang Shung, and China were invited to Tibet, and following their great gathering, their knowledge was written down and medical treatises were codified.

In the eighth century, the king of Tibet was Trisong Deutsen (742–797 CE), a very important ruler in Tibetan history. In that period lived the very famous doctor Yuthog Yönten Gönpo the Elder (708–833 CE), a descendant of Biji Gaje, the first Indian doctor who lived in Tibet. At that time doctors held another great gathering, and once more a large number of doctors came from various regions and countries, and also at that time medical treatises were composed. By this time, we have the fifty-seventh medical master of the Tibetan medical lineage, so we can see that by this time the medical tradition was already quite established.

In the late eighth century Tibetans had therefore practically gathered Asia's entire body of medical knowledge and preserved it in writing. At that same time, there lived in Tibet the great translator Vairochana, who spent a great deal of time in India, and while there he translated also texts about the two systems of Indian medicine. He too had a vision of the Medicine Buddha and put into writing the instructions he had received. He transmitted his texts to Yuthog Yönten Gönpo the Elder and hid a copy inside one of the columns of Samye, the oldest temple in Tibet. These translations of medical treatises hidden in Samye were later found by the tertön, or treasure revealer, Trapa Ngönshe, who had two main students in the field of medicine, Üpa Tatrag and Rogden, who kept the medical tradition alive.

In the sixth century, a descendant of Yuthog Yönten Gönpo the Elder was born, and was named after him, and therefore is known as Yuthog

Yönten Gönpo the Younger (1126–1202 CE). He went to India to study medicine. He had studied medicine also in Tibet and had had visions of deities that transmitted to him instructions on medicine. Inspired by these events, he compiled correct copies of all the manuscripts that constitute the foundation of Tibetan medicine. It is on his edition of the Four Tantras that the study of medicine today is based. Yuthog Yönten Gönpo the Younger was a direct descendant of Yuthog Yönten Gönpo the Elder, and he was not only a great figure in the field of medicine, but also a great yogin and siddha. He collated all of the medical traditions of his time, and with this knowledge he taught and spread widely medical science. He was not only a master of medicine, but also a meditation and dharma teacher and had as his students a great number of yogins and meditators. Three of his students continued his medical lineage, namely Trulshik, Jangpa Namgyal Dragsang (1395–1475 CE), and Zurkhar Nyamnyi Dorjee (1439–1475 CE), and a distinct medical lineage originated from each one of them. The various medical lineages became increasingly complex as each of these masters had his own disciples, who in turn had their own students, and so on.

At the time of the Fifth Dalai Lama teachers of medicine like Menrampa (Doctor of Tibetan Medicine) Sangye Gyatso (1653–1706 CE) gained particular importance and like other court doctors received the title of lha menpa, honored physician. Sangye Gyatso founded the medical college of Chagpori: greatly versed in science, he also served as regent of behalf of the Fifth Dalai Lama. Medicine was widely taught and practiced in those times, and figures like Drikung Rigdzin Chödrag, Deumar Geshe Tendzin Phuntsog, Kongtrul Yönten Gyatso, Karma Ngelek, and Ju Mipham, all residents of Eastern Tibet, became famous and respected in the entire country for their knowledge and skill in the medical field.

There are also other sources of Tibetan medicine, however. For instance, Atisha and Rinchen Sangpo, in the tenth and eleventh centuries respectively, translated texts and introduced other methods from the Indian medical tradition. Atisha taught medicine to the Four Doctors of Purang (Nyangde Senge Dra, Shaka Tri Yeshe Jungne, Ongmen Ane, and Mangmo Mentsün) in Western Tibet, and his medical tradition flourished there. Also Rinchen Sangpo, his contemporary, learned and transmitted that medical system.

At the time of the Thirteenth Dalai Lama, between the end of nineteenth and the beginning of the twentieth century, there were other famous Tibetan doctors like Champa Tubwang and his student Gyal-wang Tsultrim Nyendrup; another student was Ngawang Shar Amchi La. In 1915, under the auspices of the Thirteenth Dalai Lama, they founded Men Tsee Khang, the Medical College of Lhasa, first led by *amchi* Khyenrab Norbu (1883–1962), who had accumulated great medical knowledge as a student of Champa Tubwang, Dorgye Gyaltsen, and Jangpopa. Collating the knowledge of medicine of his times, Khyenrab Norbu was able to transmit it to his students in the Medical College of Lhasa, thus becoming the greatest driving force in spreading medical knowledge of his time. He lived until he was ninety years old.

There were, however, different medical lineages in all of Tibet – not only those centered on the king and the main figures in the country. These lineages were for the most part transmitted within one family, with the father teaching his son who in turn would teach his son, and so on for generations. Many families in Tibet transmitted medical science in this fashion. We cannot say that they were all great doctors, as great doctors are rare, but they kept medical traditions alive. Today we have a medical college in Dharamsala, in India, where students have a curriculum of theoretical and practical studies in Tibetan medicine as once people used to do in Tibet.

I spoke to you a bit about the origins of Tibetan medicine, and now I would like to explain how medicine is connected to Dharma: from this perspective, we need to consider both doctor and patient, and I will speak first about the doctor.

A patient who goes to see a doctor may or may not be an important person, and may hail from either a well to do or a poor background, but regardless of his or her social status, the patient's motivation is always their suffering. The doctor must first of all observe the condition of the patient's suffering, and upon seeing it, must regard the patient with compassion. Seeing patients suffer, looking at them with compassion, the doctor must feel love for them, a feeling that involves the will to cure them from their illness. Working with patients, trying to bring about a cure, the doctor must possess the attitude to react positively, and upon seeing them get better, must feel a spontaneous joy for this recovery. In dealing with patients, the doctor must treat them all equally, without favoring relatives or the ones he or she likes, and seeing in a bad light those he or she does not know or does not like. That is, the doctor must maintain a behavior of equality, of equanimity, towards all patients. The very act of curing a patient must be a gift, an act of generosity, and the doctor must administer the appropriate medicine, in the necessary amount, even to his poorest patient, since Tibetan doctors do not only diagnose but also provide their patients with medicines. Therefore, in the instruction to Tibetan doctors there are many indications concerning behavior that are in harmony with the instructions on the Six Perfections in the Mahayana teachings. A doctor must also possess the internal practice of both Sutra Mahayana, and Tantra. This is the way in which a doctor must relate to his patients.

We must also comprehend why, from the point of view of Dharma, a person gets sick. In Tibetan a sentient being, a subject who can move is called *semchen* – a term that indicates a being that possesses mind. Now, what is this mind that characterizes a being? Each of us has one, all beings have one: it is the sense of self, the inner sensation of the I, of oneself. Mind is what creates this sensation. If mind does not understand its true nature, it falls into illusion: this illusion, the delusion of not recognizing one's fundamental nature, constitutes basic ignorance, *marigpa*. Due to this basic ignorance, in an individual's mind the basic negative emotions, desire, aggression, and stupidity, arise. From the negative emotion of desire or attachment the humor Air originates; from the negative emotion of aggression Bile; and from stupidity Phlegm. It is from the basis of these three humors that all the various types of diseases that beings experience arise.

I have covered what I wanted to discuss with you this evening, and I will continue tomorrow speaking about the ways in which we examine an individual, their condition, and illnesses.

Venice, April 27, 1983
Morning (first session)

Moderator: Doctor Tsarong Jigme

Doctor Drolma wishes to greet everyone and to express how happy she is to participate in this conference in Venice. She asked me to read part of her biographical profile to provide some information about her life, her work, and her origins. I would like to thank on her behalf the organizers of the conference for inviting her to be part of it and for the exquisite politeness that they have shown to her so far. Then the doctor will speak to some aspects of the Tibetan medical tradition.

Doctor Lobsang Drolma was born in 1934. Her father, the governor of the Tibetan province of Kyidrog and head doctor of Khangkar, the White House Hospital, taught her the fundamentals of Tibetan medicine since childhood. Thanks to her burning desire to learn and to her capacity, when she was fourteen, she was chosen to be trained as the thirteenth representative of the unbroken family lineage of doctors in this hospital whose origin dates back to the middle of the thirteenth century. After this event, Lobsang Drolma was entrusted to the great master Pelbar Geshe Lungtog Nyima for complete and deep spiritual and practical training in the fields of Tibetan medicine and astrology. During the ensuing fifteen years she followed an intensive curriculum in which she took more than one hundred theory and practicum exams, consistently holding the first or second place among the thirty-two students in her class. She completed her studies in 1956 becoming head doctor at the Khangkar Hospital.

In the meanwhile, the Chinese had almost completed the occupation of Tibet through the strength of weapons, and all Tibetans of a certain stature and scholars were taken to China to become indoctrinated. Upon learning that the Chinese wanted to kidnap her, Lobsang Drolma escaped to India in 1959 with her family via Nepal. After a decade of extreme hardship, she was able to open her own private clinic in the very beautiful thermal station of Dalhousie. Given her increasing fame, the Tibetan government of the Dalai Lama offered her the position of head doctor of the Center of Tibetan Medicine in McLeod Ganji, near Dharamsala, where she worked for six years. Currently she supervises her own private medical institute in McLeod Ganji, where she works full time with Tibetan and Western students.

She has traveled extensively in the West and delivered lectures in prestigious cultural centers like Harvard and Yale in the USA and the Union Institute of Psychology in Switzerland.

LOBSANG DROLMA
Obstetrics and Gynecology in Tibetan medicine

I will speak about feminine diseases, obstetrics, and gynecology according to the tradition of the Tibetan medical practice. We would need more than one month to cover these topics, but today I will give a summary given our time constraints.

First of all, not all women are alike, and they can be classified in three main categories – superior, middling, and average – each of which presents specific characteristics. In the superior woman, we find eleven specific traits, and today I will talk about five of them. The first quality is a natural goodness that makes her lovable and humane with others. The second is a great love and compassion towards her parents and everyone else, that is, a quality of universal love. The third is equanimity, a balanced behavior regardless of the situation. The fourth is stability, a trait that does not diminish in any of her interactions. The fifth one is discretion, the capacity to keep to herself all secrets, anything ever told to her. These are five of her superior qualities.

The second category is the middling one. This category of women is characterized by three qualities. The first is kindness and lovingness. Unlike the superior woman, whose kindness is extended to anyone, the middling woman extends her kindness only to her relations and to those close to her. The second quality is that she knows how to please and relate to people in an altruistic way. Her third quality is the capacity to love deeply and to heal people within the sphere of her relations.

The third is the category of the ordinary or inferior woman, who does not possess any specific qualities and presents some shortcomings I will list now. The first is that she is prone to anger and to related disturbances of the mind. The second is that she easily forgets the favors and kindnesses she has received and is incapable of feeling gratitude. Her third shortcoming is that she lacks patience and the capacity to speak well of others. The fourth is insecurity and anxiety, the incapacity to face difficulties that may arise and to bear hardship. The fifth is that people tend to use her for their purposes and not to appreciate her.

These are the traits that distinguish the three different categories of women. These qualities and shortcomings do not belong only to women, also men possess them, but today's explanation pertains to women.

The characteristic aspect of female physiology is first of all the menstrual cycle, which in Tibetan medicine is divided in two categories, the bad or difficult menstrual cycle and the good one. The cycle considered bad is first of all irregular; the blood has a bad smell, and as pertains to color, the blood considered bad is dark brown or yellowish and hard to wash off. A difficult menstrual cycle is also accompanied by pain in the abdominal region and in the back. An ulterior aspect of the bad cycle is that the woman will have difficulties to conceive. In this case the woman can take medicines that will allow her to get pregnant.

A healthy menstrual cycle is regular and without pain or difficulty. The blood is red like the blood of a rabbit (this is the example used) and washes off easily. The woman who has a healthy cycle can conceive.

Conception can occur only in the presence of three elements, namely, the healthy sperm of the man, the egg of the woman, and the consciousness of the child to be born. The consciousness unites with the two other elements at the moment of conception. There are four kinds of consciousness that can enter at this juncture. The first that of an ordinary being that has no choice: it is fear that drives the consciousness towards the parents at this time.[3]

The second is that of a being who, endowed with a specific kind of consciousness, is known as an "universal ruler." This being possesses a will that allows him to travel anywhere in the universe. Within this

---

3   In the intermediate state of becoming, the deceased experience various horrific visions that drive them towards rebirth because they do not recognize them as projections of his own mind.

category there are beings with an extraordinary knowledge who are able to choose a specific birth but who later do not recall the choice made at the moment of their conception, and who, even if they have the power and the ability of choose their own birth, lose its memory after they are born. These two kinds of knowledge belong to the second category and to the "universal rulers." The third category is the consciousness of those who are at the first stage of enlightenment and that from there can move to a higher one. Even if there is an element of consciousness at the moment of conception, this kind of being later recalls little of what happened at that moment.

The fourth category is that of completely realized beings who have the power and the capacity of knowing and choosing the family and the situation in which they will be born. These beings are able to recall their previous existences, to know who and where they were before their current life, what their experiences were, and which process brought them to this existence. In the Tibetan tradition, they are called *trulku* or, in Sanskrit, *nirmanakaya*, emanations. For example, you all know that the Dalai Lama is considered a reincarnated lama; lama Namkhai Norbu too is a *trulku*, an emanation. Many lamas in the Tibetan tradition have the capacity to choose a rebirth and to know their previous experiences.

Going back to the moment of conception, at that juncture we have two specific emotions: attachment and aversion. In the Tibetan tradition, it is explained that the future male child feels attraction and attachment towards the mother and aversion and rejection towards the father, whereas the future female child feels attraction toward the father and a kind of aversion towards the mother.

At the time of conception, the consciousness of the being that is to be reborn, the father's sperm, the mother's egg, and the five elements come together to form the human being. The father's sperm has three qualities that contribute to the formation of bones, spinal cord, and in the case of a male newborn, sperm. The mother's egg provides the elements that form skin, flesh, blood, and inner organs. Based on Tibetan anatomy the five main organs are heart, lungs, kidneys, liver, and spleen. The six subsidiary organs are stomach, small intestine, gall bladder, large intestine, uterus, and bladder, all formed under the influence of the mother. The consciousness of the being forms the five sense organs, namely eyes, ears, tongue or mouth, nose, and the tactile sense of the entire body.

The five elements that form the body are *sa*, earth; *chu*, water; *me*, fire; *lung*, wind; and *namkha*, space. Their strength is not the same for everyone; it varies from person to person. The topic of elements is quite vast, and I can only give you a synthesis here. Earth has the power to solidify the parts of the body, like bones and flesh. Water has the power to give fluids to the body, lubricating and softening it. A child cannot survive without this element. Fire gives the warmth without which a person's metabolism would not work. We use the example of earth and water mixed together to make bricks: they would crumble without heat. So, the fire element allows earth and water to combine. Wind has the characteristic of movement, and creates it. It goes through the blood vessels and channels and is eliminated from pores and various bodily orifices. *Namkha*, space, constitutes the space in which the fetus will grow: without space the fetus would not be able to grow, to move, and would not survive. In astrology wood replaces wind, and metal, space, but in medicine they are interchangeable.

Gestation lasts thirty-eight weeks: the process of formation of the newborn should be completed in the tenth month. All throughout the entire period from conception to birth, the powers of specific winds or *lung* act in the body and allow the unfolding of certain processes in precise moments in the nine months of pregnancy. Let us mention a few of these processes that take place during the embryo's development. One of the first signs of conception is that menstruations cease during the first month. It is also possible that this would be due to disease, but it could also be a sign of conception.

The first power of the wind is called *sogdzin*. Its power and function are to combine the five elements and the three constituents [consciousness, sperm, and egg] that unite at the moment of conception. In the second week, the lung is called *kuntu düpa*; the force of this wind travels in the embryo through the semen and blood of the parents. It is said that at this time the sperm and egg combined resemble gelatin.

The wind of the third week is called *zökha* (*bzod dka'*), and the embryo looks round and white like thick curd or yoghurt. Up to this moment the sex of the fetus is not yet determined: during the third week, it is still possible to choose it, or in effect, to change it with specific medicines or invocations. In India many people believe that having a son is important for their survival, and the process to change the sex of the fetus or to decide its gender is achieved successfully, but for us Tibetans there is no difference between having a daughter or a son.

By the fifth week, the fetus has already undergone many changes: head and limbs become visible and many other parts have already come into being, like the umbilical cord, which is said is like four conjoined petals. Once the umbilical cord is formed, it is important for the mother to eat properly because now the food she eats goes to the child through it. It is also important for the pregnant woman to rest, to avoid hard work, to keep a healthy diet, and not to ingest medicines to expel parasites from the body because it could be harmful. She needs to be careful not to fall, to avoid any accident, and not to strain her body in any way because it could damage the fetus's senses. To avoid the possibility of miscarriage, the mother needs to follow the doctor's advice on diet and behavior beneficial to the child.

During the fifth week, the central part of the umbilical cord is connected to the sixteen vertebrae of the spinal cord whose development progresses from the umbilical cord upwards. The connection between the central part and the spinal cord takes place when the development of the upper part gets to the heart.

During the sixth week, according to Tibetan medicine, *uma*, the central channel connected to long life, comes into being; the vital air goes through it and reaches the center of the body. In this period, winds traverse the channels (veins, arteries, and so on) that have already formed in the body.

In the seventh week, once the navel chakra and the heart chakra have formed, there is a gap equivalent to sixteen fingers of the baby between the heart and the throat chakra in this upwards process of formation.

The belly center is said to correspond to the dharmakaya, and the throat chakra to the samboghakaya. The throat chakra is a very important point, and it is quite dangerous if it becomes damaged. It is connected to the first vertebra. In this period, the mother must pay a lot of attention to the positions she takes and she must avoid any incident because everything that happens to her damages directly to the child. She must also pay attention to her diet: for example, eating a lot of pork, aside from harming the mother, can have negative effects on the sense organs and the intelligence of the child, and anything that happens to the mother's body directly affects the child.

During the eighth week, the internal development moves towards the head. It is said that the distance between the throat chakra and the head chakra corresponds to fourteen fingers of the baby. During this period *uma*, the central channel, reaches the top of the head and then comes down to a point between the eyes, which in the Tibetan tradition is called wisdom eye or third eye.

In the ninth month, the child is ready for birth: he or she feels a great discomfort, smells the bad odor of the uterus, feels entrapped, and has an urge to go out. This is the beginning of the birth profess. Often, during the ninth month, there is a lot of movement inside the uterus: the baby kicks and moves a lot because of the inclination and the urgency to come out. At this point the strength of the *lung* called *thursel* takes over, and helps the baby turn in the uterus until his head turns downwards, and the child is pushed downwards, towards the cervix. There are three phases in the dilatation of the cervix: the initial opening, the dilatation, and finally the opening that allows the head to go through. There are three possible positions for the head of the baby: high, sideways, and low. If the head is low there will be no problems, and the birth can take place without the doctor's help. If the head is still high, the doctor must intervene to turn the child as to ease the birth process. If the head is sideways, the mother will notice it by herself: this can create great problems.

Moderator:

Thank you very much, Doctor Drolma. Unfortunately we need to stop here as we have run out of time; we will continue tomorrow.

TROGAWA RINPOCHE
Pulse Diagnosis

In Tibetan medicine, we use three principal methods to diagnose illness: pulse analysis, urine analysis, and examination of the tongue. Let us begin with pulse analysis. Considering the relation between the patient, his pulse, and the doctor, we see the pulse as the messenger that brings information about the patient to the doctor. In pulse analysis we need to consider thirteen factors:

1. Preliminaries.
2. The best time for pulse analysis.
3. The point in which we take the pulse.
4. The pressure of the fingers on the pulse, i.e. the pressure exerted by the fingers to measure the pulse.
5. The interpretation of the pulse and of the information derived from the exam.
6. The natural condition of the pulse, i.e. the pulse of a healthy person.
7. The season that is the pulse variation in the course of the four seasons, spring, summer, fall, and winter. We consider pulse analysis in relationship to the Five Elements and the Four Relations. The five elements in this case are connected to astrology and are Earth, Metal, Water, Wood, and Fire. The four relations are mother, son, friend, and enemy. This is how we conduct pulse analysis in connection with astrology.

8. This is the special category called the "seven wondrous pulses." This category is based on the natural pulse and involves seven factors. This is the method through which doctors can make prophecies by examining the pulse.
9. This is the method by which the doctor differentiates between a healthy pulse and sickly one.
10. This is the precise method by which the doctor identifies the illness of the patient.
11. The death pulse, that is, how we can establish when a person is about to die and why.
12. The demonic pulse: by this examination, one can establish which negative influence of the outside environment has struck the patient, where it came from, its characteristics, and its effects.
13. The last factor is called "pulse of the strength of the individual," and through this exam one can establish how long a person will live.

This is what we must understand when we study the pulse.

1. Preliminaries

Let us examine these thirteen categories beginning with the preliminaries. One or two days before the pulse is examined, the patient will have to pay attention to his diet and physical activities. He should avoid food that overheats the body, like eating too much meat or drinking too much alcohol; he should also avoid the food, and especially the liquids, that have too much cooling effect. The question of meat is more complex because not all different kinds of meat have the same characteristics, as some heat and some cool the body. Meats that heat the body are, for example, yak, poultry, or horse. Also, fish is a type of meat that has heating effects. Goat and pork both have a cooling effect. One must also avoid foods that are hard to digest.

Before the pulse exam one must avoid activities that are too intense. For instance, one should not eat and then immediately go to sleep. One should also avoid excessive physical exercise, sunbathing for too long, or doing hard work because these activities disturb the body. If one is too relaxed or too excited the right conditions to measure the pulse are lacking. One should not change one's sleeping habits, and should instead go to bed at the usual time, without sleeping too much or too little. One should also avoid talking too much: it is positive to avoid worries, overthinking, and fixating on problems.

These, when it is possible, are the preliminary conditions necessary for the pulse examination. Sometimes it happens that a patient will need to be examined immediately without time to conduct all the preliminaries to ensure an optimal pulse. In this instance one tries to intervene in the best way, for example, by having the patient rest a little bit before taking the pulse.

2. Time

When is it best to take one's pulse? The right moment is dawn, when the first rays of light hit the sky and have not yet touched the earth, and ideally the patient will still be in bed, that is, before altering the body by getting up, and before ingesting any drink or food or engaging in any activity. And why is it best to take the pulse just at the boundary between day and night? Because the forces of the day's heat and the night's coolness in that very moment are very balanced in the environment.

3. Place

Thirdly, we must think about the place where we measure the pulse, and we do so right under the "sign of the bracelet." Every person has a line around the wrist, and there are people who have more than one. We take the pulse two fingers from the first line, on the side of the thumb, with three fingers. The point in which the doctor positions their thumb, on the opposite side of the wrist in correspondence with the position of their little finger, is very important, because to put the thumb on the back of the hand disturbs the pulse. When you take the pulse you should never put the patient's elbow on a hard surface or pull up their sleeve in such a way that it constricts the arm.

In Tibetan, the index finger is called *dzubmo*, or pointy finger, while the middle finger is called *kungmo,* or central finger, and the ring finger is called *sinlag*. Why do we have to take the pulse in this specific point, beginning exactly two fingers below the pulse's bracelet? Because when we touch the radial artery we are neither too close or too far from the heart. As a matter of fact, if we wanted to take the pulse very close to the source, we should do so on the side of the neck, where the pulse is quite strong, but this is difficult because it is too close to the heart, so what we feel is the heart's pulse, and nothing much more. It is very hard to distinguish the subtleties of the pulse when you are close to the heart. For example, two people who stand at the opposite sides of a waterfall and try to have a conversation will not be able to communicate because of the noise, and the effect is similar if one tries to take the pulse on the side of the neck.

You can also measure the pulse far away from the source, far from the heart, for example on the top of the foot, but if we do that, we are too far from the heart, and the transmission of the message of the body is lost. To take the pulse in the foot is like receiving a message from someone coming from far away: the message is partially true and partially false, and in the end, quite confused. Taking the pulse on the foot is a little like that. The pulse on the hand, instead, is neither too far nor too close. It is a bit like what in Tibet we call "screaming distance," about five hundred spans; one span being the distance between thumb and the little finger when you spread your fingers. From that distance, if you scream, you can be heard. Why is it so important to take the pulse in this place? The radial artery is like a freeway, a main road taken by everybody. The relationship between prana, or the energy of the body, and blood is like a businessman that manages to know what is happening everywhere: who bought what, who sold what, and what is happening business-wise in other places. In the radial artery of the pulse, blood pressure and the blood reflect the conditions of the entire body.

We examine the pulse with three fingers of the right hand and three of the left hand. Every finger has two positions, the right and left side of the finger itself. These twelve positions are called *patse* in ancient Tibetan. Usually the doctor takes the patient's right pulse with the left hand, and the left pulse with the right hand, but the pulse of the "life force" – *la* or protective energy – the doctor takes with the right hand on the right pulse of the patient, in the lower part of the palm's surface of the pulse, on the ulnar artery, on the side of the left finger, between the tendons.

To examine the "pulse of death" in order to discover if a person is about to die and why exactly, we must first of all understand that when a person dies the elements are reabsorbed one within the other. To understand if this is what is happening, you need to examine in the foot's pulse, in a point called *böltsa*, that is the dorsal artery of the foot.

4. Pressure

Let us turn now to the pressure we apply to take the pulse. With our index finger we lightly touch the pulse, barely brushing against the skin. With the middle finger we push a bit more on the pulse so that we lightly put pressure on the flesh. With your ring finger you push until you touch the bone. Why do we need to use different levels of pressure? As we move from the wrist to the elbow the arm becomes heavier, more solid: going instead towards the hand the arm becomes thinner. Since the arm is shaped like a turnip, we put different levels of pressure on the pulse to conform to the arm's shape.

5. Interpretation of the pulse

How do we take the pulse, exactly? First of all the doctor should have very sensitive and soft fingers, without calluses or wounds. There needs to be thermal balance between the doctor and the patient: if they are both either too cold or too hot it is not possible to measure the pulse in an appropriate way, because both parties need to be balanced in terms of heat and cold. Let us imagine the patient is male.

To treat a male patient, we begin by examining the left pulse. We examine it with the index of the right hand, which has two positions. The external position [i.e., towards the thumb] indicates the heart's pulse. The internal position [towards the middle finger] indicates the condition of the small intestine. The position of the middle finger towards the index finger indicates the spleen, and towards the ring finger the stomach. The external position of the ring finger, towards the middle finger, indicates the left kidney; the internal position indicates what in Tibetan we call *samseu*: the gonads for men, and the uterus and the ovaries in women.

Taking the right pulse with the left hand, the external side of the index finger indicates the condition of the lungs, while the internal one indicates the condition of the descending colon. The external side of the middle finger indicates the condition of the liver, and the internal one pancreas, bile, and gall bladder. The side of the ring finer towards the middle finger indicates the right kidney and the left side, towards the little finger, indicates the bladder. These are the positions to read the condition of the various organs if the patient is male.

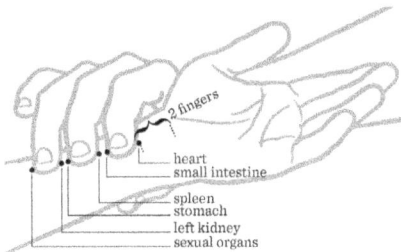

Left pulse of the male patient, right hand of the doctor

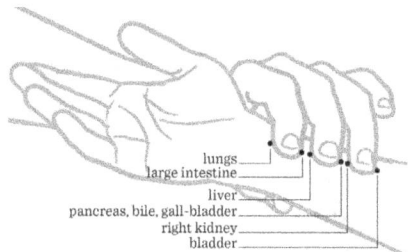

Right pulse of the female patient, left hand of the doctor

Figure 2. Taking the pulse in male and female patients

With a woman, the doctor begins by reading the right pulse with the left hand. We must remember that in a woman the pulses of heart and lungs are reversed because the position of the heart is slightly different: in women the heart points to the right, and in men towards the left. In Tantra, they say that women have the nature of transcendental knowledge, and this is indicated in the fact that their heart points to the right. Men have the nature of method and their heart points to the left. All the other pulses are read in the same positions for men and women; only the positions of heart and lungs are reversed.

6. The pulse of a healthy person

Let us move on to the next category, which is the pulse of a normal and healthy individual. There are three general typologies of pulse for normal and healthy people. They are called *potsa*, *motsa*, and *changchub semtsa*, meaning, male, female, and natural pulse respectively. At times you can find, however, a male pulse mixed with a neutral one, and this also happens with a female pulse. The neutral pulse sometimes appears on its own. The woman with a male pulse will have a child. The man with a female pulse will live a long life. The men or women who have a true neutral pulse will live long and without disease. The neutral pulse is called this way when we encounter it in normal people, while in people of high spiritual level we call it the "bodhisattva pulse," or the pulse of enlightened mind, and we find it not only among great lamas, but also among dakinis. If we have a neutral pulse, the people who are our superiors will be good and kind to us, while those in an inferior position will be harsh. Those who have a neutral pulse have awful relationships with the uncles, aunts, and other family members who will turn against them and become hostile. The person who truly has a neutral pulse, without any male or female characteristic, cannot have children. An example of a truly neutral pulse is Milarepa. If in a family, let us say the father, has a male pulse, and the other, let us say the mother, has a neutral pulse, thanks to the strength of the male pulse the couple could have children, but since the woman has a neutral pulse, there will be no offspring. If one of the partners has a female pulse and the other has a neutral pulse, for sure the couple will not have male children, but only one daughter. If both partners have a male pulse, in the majority of cases, the children will be males; similarly, if both have female pulses in the great majority of cases daughters will be born. To be able to determine all of this we must examine the pulses of the family members when they are healthy.

7. *Effects of the seasons*

The seventh category deals with the effects of the four seasons. In order to understand spring, we need to consider the pulse of the liver. Keeping in mind that spring lasts ninety days, if we subtract the last eighteen days, we are left with seventy-two days, and this is the period of the pulse of the liver. The element of spring is wood. During the period of the element wood, all plants, herbs, and so on grow (at least in Tibet, I am not sure that elsewhere is the same). There is a constellation[4] in particular called in Tibetan *taba* (*brta pa*, Regulus), which begins in the first Tibetan month. In the second month in the sky we find the constellation wö (*dbo*, Leo). In the third month there is the constellation *nagpa* (*nag pa*, Virgo), the black star. These three constellations, which reach their zenith at midnight, indicate the first three months of the year. Starting from the thirteenth day of the third month, the last eighteen days are the period of the pulse of the spleen. This period marks the end of spring and the first appearance of the nightingale in Tibet. As a matter of fact, the last eighteen days of each season are the period of the pulse of the spleen.

Summer is the period of the pulse of the heart. That is the natural pulse, the pulse that goes with the period of the year. This season's element is fire, therefore spring's predominant element is wood, and that of summer is fire. At times in Tibetan texts one finds the word *shingtse* (*shing rtse*), which literally means "tip of the wood," but in this context, connected to spring, it means pulse of the element wood. In summer in Tibet leaves grow on trees and plants, and it rains more often. The constellation of the fourth month is called *saga* (*sa ga*, Libra), that of the fifth month is called *non* (*snron*, Antares), and that of the sixth month is called high water, *chutöd* (*chu stod*, Sagittarius). These three constellations, which reach their respective zenith at midnight, indicate the three months of summer. Thus the first seventy-two days of summer constitute the period of activity of the fire pulse of the heart. The rest of the period constitutes

---

4   Tib. *rgyu skar*, Sanskr. *nakṣatra*: of these lunar mansions some are constellations, whereas others are single stars or, like Regulus, multiple star systems.

the time of the spleen pulse, and like in springtime, Summer is the time of pigeons because in Tibet you can hear them coo all summer long.

The third period is autumn: this is the time of maturation, when wheat and everything else brings fruit. This is harvest time, the fruit on the trees is ripe, and so on. In this time, we have the pulse of the lungs. The element of autumn is metal. The metal pulse of the lungs lasts seventy-two days, the first seventy-two days of autumn. The constellations of autumn are *droshin* (*gro bzhin*, Eagle), *trumtöd* (*khrums stod*, Pegasus), and *yupa* (*dbyu ga*, Aries). These are the constellations reaching their respective zenith at midnight during the fall months. This period is called the time of bird flocks. In Tibet, the wrens land in the fields to collects the seeds left over after the harvest, and as they fly away they make a characteristic noise that one doesn't hear in other periods of the year when the wrens do not fly in flocks.

In the three winter months the earth and also the lakes freeze. The natural pulse of winter is that of the kidneys. The element of this period is water. This period, like the others, also lasts seventy-two days. The last eighteen days we have the fourth pulse of the spleen. In the tenth month, the constellation at the zenith is *mindrug* (*smin drug*, Taurus). In the eleventh month it is *go* (*mgo*, Orion), and in the twelfth it is called *gyal* (*rgyal*, Cancer). These constellations indicate respectively the tenth, eleventh, and twelfth Tibetan month.

7.1 The Five Elements and the Four Relationships

Now we must also consider the relationships of mother, son, friend, and foe in relation to *shing, me, sa, chag, chu*, that is, wood, fire, earth, metal, and water. We will try to briefly cover this topic. Let us consider the five elements in the hand: wood corresponds to the thumb, fire to the index, earth to the middle finger, metal to the ring finger, and water to the little finger. But perhaps with this diagram (see Diagram number 3) it is easier to understand. The child of wood is fire; the child of fire is earth; the child of earth is metal; and the child of metal is water. The relationship is cyclical, so the child of water is wood. In reverse order:

the mother of water is metal; the mother of metal is earth; the mother of earth is fire; the mother of fire is wood.

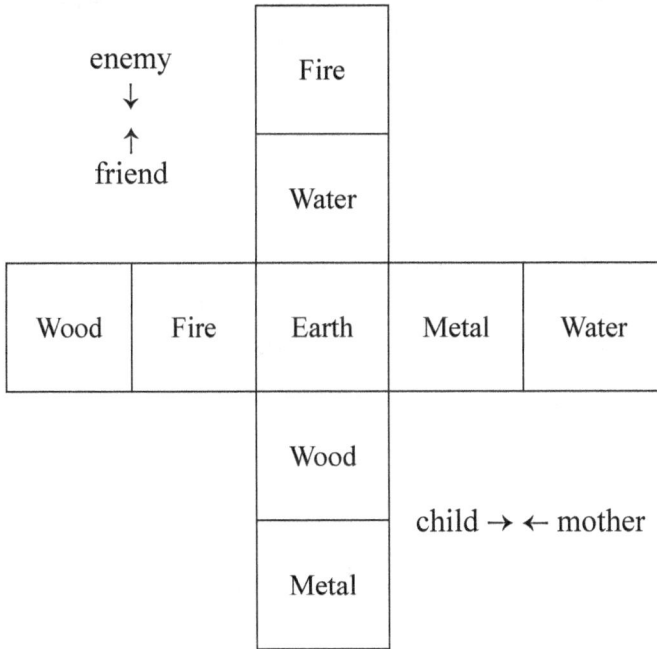

	Fire		
enemy ↓ ↑ friend	Water		

Wood	Fire	Earth	Metal	Water

	Wood	
	Metal	child → ← mother

Figure 3. The child-parent relation between different elements

The above diagram should be read as follows: fire is the child of wood, metal is the mother of water, water is the enemy of fire, wood is the friend of metal, and so forth.

This is the way to establish the mother/child relationship. We the have the following sequence: fire, water, earth, wood, metal. The enemy of fire is water; the enemy of water is earth; the enemy of earth is wood; the enemy of wood is metal; and the enemy of metal is fire; and this is the way the cycle of enemies works.

Now let us look at the cycle of friends. The friend of metal is wood; the friend of wood, earth; that of earth, water; the friend of water, fire;

and that of fire, metal. Thus this is the way we establish friends and foes, mothers and children. In this graphic the earth is at the center. In the seventh category we find the various characteristics of the various pulses that indicate a variety of situations.

8. The Seven Wondrous Pulses

Now we will turn to the eighth topic, namely the seven wondrous pulses, which should be taken when the body is at peace and in a calm state. Being able to read them requires a specific way and practice called *namgyi*, a sort of divination technique that reads omens based on the pulse. Here we have seven subdivisions of topics:

a. The first is called "the condition of one's home" (*khyim phyva*) and concerns family members; it is possible to foresee the existence of obstacles or specific problems that hinder or could hinder family members, their successes and failures, and so on and so forth.
b. The second wondrous pulse (*mgrong phyva*) allows us to learn when family members on the road will come back, and if we should expect guests and visitors.
c. The third (*dgra phyva*) deals with war. In ancient times in Tibet an *amchi* always traveled with the army, and he or she would be able, by reading the commander's pulse right before combat, to predict whether the attack against the enemy (or vice versa) would succeed or fail. In other words, if one is worried about an enemy attack, there is another pulse to determine the outcome. In Tibet, we use the word *par gol* (*phar rgol*) to mean "attack," and *tsur gol* (*tshur rgol*) to mean "to be attacked."
d. The fourth wondrous pulse concerns business and money (*grogs phyva*). Through the reading of the pulse an *amchi* can discern if a person will be successful in business, if they will make money, if they will become rich or poor, and so on. In Eastern Tibet, where nomads rear cattle, they use this pulse a lot to know what will

happen to the animals, if they will increase in number, or if they will have problems.

e. The fifth wondrous pulse is called *dön cha* (*gdon phyva*), an ancient Tibetan word that refers to the negative influences coming from the surrounding environment. The reading of this pulse allows the amchi to establish which negative influences can hit a person, where they come from, and which kind they belong to. And there are many kinds indeed.

f. The sixth pulse is called "fire and water reversed" (*me chu go ldog*) and refers to the practice to take the pulse of one person to diagnose the illness of somebody else. For instance, if a father and son are separated from a great distance, the one between the two who wants to know the condition of the other asks the *amchi* to take his pulse, which, from the father's pulse, will be able to determine whether the son is ill, or vice versa: and if he is ill, which sickness it is, and whether it can be cured, and how serious it is. This can also be done between mother and daughter, and between wife and husband to learn what is happening to the person who is far away.

g. The seventh wondrous pulse is related with pregnant women (*bu rtsa*). From this pulse, we can understand whether the child brings benefit to the family, if the mother is going to have health problems or issues in her relationship with the baby.

Sometimes when we take the wondrous pulses, we must use the mother/child and friend/foe relationships; in other cases, it is not necessary to use them. And this is all I wanted to say in relationship to the seven wondrous pulses.

9. Difference between a healthy and unhealthy pulse

The ninth category helps us determine if a person is healthy or ill. In order to establish this, there are two basic conditions through which we take the pulse. The first is related to the *amchi*'s breathing, and the second has to do with the characteristics of the pulse. The Tibetan medical texts are very ancient, dating back two to three thousand years ago, and because there were no clocks at that time people used the *amchi*'s natural breathing to measure time. So if the pulse frequency is equal to five beats every three and a half seconds, the person being diagnosed is healthy. A higher frequency indicates fever or a heat-related illness. If the pulse frequency is six beats every three and a half seconds, the fever is low, but if it rises to seven, eight, or nine beats, it means that the fever is increasingly higher; if it gets to ten beats, there is not much to do. If there are four beats every three and a half seconds, the body [temperature] will be slightly cool; if there are three beats the body [temperature] will be low; if there are only two beats, we have a serious illness connected to coolness. With only one beat every three and a half seconds there is very little left to do. Therefore the first thing Tibetan doctors do when they take the pulse is to count the pulse beats in relationship to one's own breathing: about five beats mean that the patient is basically healthy.

Thereafter we must consider the pulse aspect and all its characteristics, and in this way we will discover possible problems. Some problems related to the pulse exist since birth, meaning that the patient has always had them, and therefore one should not give them too much importance. On the other hand, the presence of variations in the places where a person usually has a normal pulse – for instance, a heavier or lighter pulse, with a different characteristic from the one the patient had when healthy – points to the presence of an illness. Therefore, the *amchi* visiting a patient for the first time has difficulty in establishing exactly their condition. In order to be able to pronounce a correct diagnosis, the *amchi* needs to know the person, otherwise, not knowing that specific person's pulse when they are healthy, it is not easy to diagnose an illness on the basis of changes in the pulse. For example, we usually have three kinds of pulses: male, female, and neutral. The variations towards any of these pulses are symptoms of illness in one person and a sign of health in another.

Thus, diagnosis is much harder if we do not know the pulse of a person when they are healthy. There are many natural variations of the pulse that simply indicate the characteristics of an individual and not the presence of illness. There are people with a strong and dynamic pulse and those with a very weak one. For some the pulse beat moves to the side of their arm. Some have curious gaps in which one cannot feel anything, but this is the natural flow of their pulse and not a symptom of illness. So, during the first visit, the *amchi* asks many questions, and the first question is about the natural condition of the pulse. Then the *amchi* asks if the pulse has irregularities, which means if another *amchi*, for example, has in the past told the patient that certain irregularities are normal in their pulse. The *amchi* will be able to take the pulse without difficulties if the patient is able to answer that they do not have natural irregularities and that they have a male or female or neutral pulse.

10. Identifying the disease

The tenth topic relates to identifying illness. We can divide this topic in two sections: general and specific considerations. The specific considerations concern heat and cold. We have six types of pulses that point to illnesses of warm nature or fever and six types that relate to sicknesses with a cold nature. When we take the pulse in order to identify the illness, there are two important things to keep in mind, namely the strength of the pulse and the feeling we get when our three fingers touch each hand in the prescribed points. In terms of pulse strength, we need to keep in mind the effect that the various conditions of the three humors (air, bile, and phlegm) exert on it. The air pulse resembles a ball floating on water, so the doctor feels something like a little ball moving on the surface. You can feel it when you take the pulse with a very light pressure, but if you push hard, it disappears, you cannot feel it anymore. The bile pulse resembles entangled horse-hair: it feels narrow and rigid to the touch. The phlegm pulse is like a slow, loose, and twisted thread of wool. I would also like to mention the blood pulse that is coarse and rough and that, like the air pulse, disappears when pressure is applied. Nowadays people are afraid of blood illnesses, especially high blood pressure.

In the west people do not differentiate among the different types of high blood pressure. We have two types, of which only one is real, because it presents the four heats that we expect in this condition. The second kind is not connected to heat but to the element air. The air and blood pulse without heat is coarse and rough, and when you apply pressure it persists, it does not disappear.

Air, bile, and phlegm are the three fundamental humors of the body and relate one to the other. I will speak first of all of the relationship between air and bile. As I have already said, when you take the pulse on the surface, you will feel the bile pulse like horsehair tightly braided. If you push, the pulse persists; you can still feel it, and this means that there is a joined condition of air and bile.

Now we will talk about air and phlegm together. Let us now see what happens when we have air and phlegm together. The condition of phlegm, if you touch lightly the pulse, feels smooth, and if you push, no matter how much, you can still feel it clearly. If we consider bile and phlegm together, when you take the pulse pushing lightly, on the surface you will feel the condition of phlegm, smooth, and when you push you can feel bile, rigid like a bundle of horsehair tightly bound. Then we have the pulse of glandular secretions that vibrate in the pulse. They are very peculiar and recognizable because they seem to pulse with difficulty.

In the pulse, you can also feel the presence of parasites. In this case the pulse will be very tense and with knots, like a rope sealing a sack. At times, you feel a pulse that goes flat: this too indicates the presence of parasites. At times, we encounter leprosy. Which pulse does it have? With leprosy, the pulse appears to hesitate; not only does it hesitate, it also vibrates in various ways. There are also pulses that indicate various malaises in the body. In these cases, the pulse becomes heavy and seems to bounce.

There is also a condition called dark phlegm that denotes an illness cause by a disorder of air, bile, phlegm, and blood all together. The pulse is big and strong, and also feels very full. The weakest point, however, of this pulse is under the middle finger. There are many pulses that indicate bodily conditions caused by trauma, accidents, falls, and so on.

In the case of incidents, the pulse tends to be subtle, and deep down we can find characteristics that indicate an illness of a cool nature. How is the pulse of a person who has had a fever for a short time? In the first phase of the fever the pulse is subtle and very quick, and, in this case, we give medication. When the fever is fully developed the pulse is stronger, and the curve shows that the growth of the fever shows three or four notable characteristics. If the fever is very high in the pulse, we find five characteristics: when all five are present, the cure is very challenging. There is a sixth characteristic of fever in the pulse, and when all six are present there is no hope of recovery. If we do not apply the right remedy in time, when the fever is not yet fully developed, there is the risk of a problematic fever. With this pulse, if you push lightly you still can feel the fever, but underneath it you can feel a second pulse moving quite rapidly.

We have the "danger pulse" that indicates an infectious condition. It is a very distinct pulse, which feels like a knot, and as if you had two pulses beating together. We call them brother and sister pulses in Tibetan, and what this means is that we have two very thin pulses beating together instead of only one.

Then we have the pulse that indicates that a person has been wounded. This pulse is heavy and large, that is rounded, but this latter characteristic can be felt only if you can find and feel this pulse. There is also something fast to this pulse.

Poisons too have different influences and effects on the pulse. We have a basic pulse that shows a person has been poisoned: it is rough and we call it *punpa*, a word used only for the characteristic and the type of this pulse; we can understand its meaning only when we feel it. Then we have the meat poison: the pulse is thin, fast, and has a specific aspect, but it is hard to recognize, and until we have a lot of experience we can confuse it with other kinds. The pulse that indicates meat poison has four precise characteristics, and this is why we can mistake it for other pulses.

Now if a person falls and hits her head, we want to know if she has received any damage, like a cranial fracture or brain damage – any head wound. We also want to know if there is damage to any other organ because of the fall, especially damage to the kidneys. These are considerations related to heat illnesses or with fever. In fever-related sickness, we also need to consider factors such as malnourishment, lack of heat to the stomach, problems with glandular secretions, and so on.

This is a synthesis, just to give you an idea, of the way we examine and take the pulse, and of what an *amchi* feels when they diagnose a disease. To pinpoint exactly what and where a disease is, recognizing its characteristics is the second part of identifying an illness in the pulse. The *amchi* recognizes the illnesses of the upper part of the body with the middle finger, of the central part of the body with the middle finger, and of the lower part of the body, especially of the kidneys, with the ring finger. We have examined some aspects and perceptions of the pulse. Using three fingers the *amchi* not only examines the pulse they feel, but also its exact location, and on this basis they can identify the illness in the corresponding body part. Then you need to consider if we feel the pulse on the external or internal side of the finger, in order to identify the disease better.

11. Death Pulse

Now I will speak about the eleventh category, that of death and the conditions that lead to death. There are three points to take in consideration. The first is a change in the character of the pulse, which is different from when the person is in good health, but it is not that of a sick person. We thus speak of a change in the basic character of the pulse.

The second thing to consider in the death pulse is its lack: the pulse is incomplete, and this indicates imminent death. We can also find signs in the sense organs, in the tongue, eyes, ears, which seem to lose their shine, and this is visible from the outside. Furthermore, their functions also seem to decline. We have five organs considered meaningful parts of the body: heart, lungs, liver, spleen, and kidneys. The inner flower of the heart blooms on the tongue [meaning that the symptom manifests on the tongue]; the flower of the lungs blooms on the nose; the flower of the liver blooms in the eyes; the flower of the spleen blooms on the mouth; and the flower of the kidneys blooms in the ears. When the person is about to die, these flowers and the basic organs change their characteristics.

The third characteristic of the death pulse is that it is lasting. We have three lasting pulses: in specific illnesses, in a dying person, and in the presence of a negative external influence. It is easy to mix them up, and therefore we need to learn how to differentiate one from the other.

12. The demonic pulse

The twelfth category includes negative external influences and their diagnosis through the pulse. There are five characteristics based on external influences, or, if you prefer, on the demonic pulse. The pulse under demonic influences changes constantly, and changes in different ways – it stops irregularly, at times it stops and then starts again, it seems to have a double beat.

When we spoke of the seven wondrous pulses we mentioned the pulses that indicate negative external influences, to the point that we can determine exactly which negative external influence is affecting the person and from whence it comes. The pulse has five basic character-istics that can indicate an external influence, and we need to feel and pinpoint with precision where, in the three fingers, we feel this pulse. If the amchi, using the left hand on the right hand pulse of a male patient feels a demonic pulse under his index finger, it means that the external influence is affecting the lungs. This means that we are dealing with demonic influence of a naga, a black naga that thus hails from the West.[5]

We can detect which negative influence is affecting a person among the many possible, and also which direction it comes from – i.e., east, north, west, or south, or in between directions, meaning northeast, northwest, southeast, southwest – and which organ is affected. We then need to understand why the person is receiving this influence; if it is

---

5   Nagas are one of the eight classes of powerful beings that cause illnesses.

because of something they own, or because they dug some earth, moved boulders, or bathed in a certain river, for example.[6]

If the illness is related to something we own, for example, we need to understand exactly which is the object that is causing the problem. For this reason, in Tibet people worry a lot about ancient objects and their property in general, like for instance, old inheritances coming from monasteries. Western people instead love antiques. What matters in the end, is what one believes in, I suppose. So today I gave you one more reason to worry! [The audience laughs.]

Another way to discover an illness consists in understanding which organ or part of the body is troubled. When the external negative influence has been identified, the *amchi* needs to discover which ritual can remove it, and then prescribes formulas to recite and rituals to be performed in accordance with the customs of religious tradition of the patient.

13. The pulse of the la (bla), an individual's vital force

Among of the six categories of sentient beings, we belong to that of human beings. We all have something that indicates the length of our life, and this something is called *la* (*bla*). This is a very ancient concept that dates back to the first period of Tibetan history, when Bön was the main tradition. Back then, *la* was already well known and was considered as a sort of individual characteristic made up by light and darkness. This is in a way the story of its origins. Now, in adherence with related teaching and to the medical treatises, a person has three types of pulse that indicate the length of one's life. The first permeates the entire body: it is a sort of *la* made of light and is capable of moving and relocating from one place to another. The second pulse of life moves from within towards the outside of the body together with the breath. The first, the pulse that moves with the la, moves from one place to another in various parts of the body, and one can even cal-

---

6   In Tibetan lore construction works that greatly alter the nature of a place and that upset the natural environment, like leveling mountains, deviating rivers, digging deep in the earth, are considered negative and as harbingers of disasters.

culate its exact position.[7] The pulse or energy that moves with one's breath, moves from within to outside the body and gets as far as about twelve fingers in front of one's face. There is a lot more to say on life and vital force, and I hope we will have time to explore this topic more before the end of the conference.

When we take the *la* pulse – which, I remind you, we take in a specific point on the arm – this changes at a certain moment. From the moment it changes, there is a method to count the pulse, connected to breathing, which indicates the vital force left in a person. There are also methods to read omens from the *la* pulse that depend on how the pulse manifests, from the aspect that it assumes when you take it. We have thus deepened a bit the reading of the pulse as diagnosis, and this is part of the thirteenth category of pulse reading.

In Tibetan medicine, to analyze the condition of an individual we also use urine and tongue analysis and we ask the patient questions. If we have enough time, tomorrow or the day after, I would like to continue to speak about diagnostic methods.

Moderator

I thank Trogawa Rinpoche for this in-depth and well-structured presentation on the pulse. I just would like to add that this topic comes from the *Gyüzhi, The Four Tantras*. This gives you an idea of the precision with which the entire manuscript is organized. And what we heard relates only to the pulse. The first, second, third, and fourth Tantra fit one into the other perfectly as a whole: it is a fascinating text, and I hope that one day someone will be able to translate it in its entirety. I believe that already in 1840 or thereabout the Russian Czar commissioned its translation, and since then people have been trying to translate. I really hope we can collaborate and translate it; it is really important.

---

7   You can refer to the Tibetan calendar prepared by Chögyal Namkhai Norbu and published every year by Shang Shung Publications.

Venice, April 27, 1983
Afternoon (first session)

Moderator:

Professor Namkhai Norbu will give a presentation on incurable diseases like cancer.

NAMKHAI NORBU
Working with incurable diseases

I will now explain about illnesses that are hard to cure, as planned, but I think that first of all it is useful to learn how Tibetan medicine understands illness, and how main diseases arise and which kind of diseases we have. As the other doctors and I have explained both yesterday and today, the principle of illness is based on what we call the three humors or *duwa* – which means the potentiality, the force that sustains life – namely *lung, tripa,* and *peken.* When circumstances, such as behavior, diet, or the function of an individual's energy, disturb the humors, what we call illness manifests. The illness can be singular, that is, typical of *lung*/Air, *tripa*/Bile (in the West people refer to liver, but in this case these two terms are synonymous), or of *peken*/Phlegm; or it can be conjoined, for instance we can have a *lung* illness conjoined with a *tripa* illness, or a *tripa* one conjoined with a *peken* one. In Tibetan a principal illness conjoined with another is called *denpa (ldenpa)*, which means conjoined illness.

Then we have the illnesses we call *duwa*, in which all three humors are equally unbalanced. In this group, we find illnesses with two different characteristics: the actual *duwa* illnesses caused by disturbances of all three humors, and another group of illnesses that manifests in another way and that we called *lanyen (bla gnyan)* in Tibetan. What does this mean? *La* means supreme. For example, with *lama* we mean a teacher, someone we consider supreme. Another meaning of *la* is the condition of the vital force of a person. If in a person the function of life force is not regular, or, as I explained yesterday morning, if the positive force is diminished or weakened, we say that their *la* is weakened. Especially in the ancient Bönpo tradition there was a ritual to strengthen the *la*, or to call it back to the individual when it went missing. This very common ritual existed not only in that tradition a long time ago, but it is still used today also in Tibetan Buddhism because it is very useful. *La* is sometimes translated with soul, but it does not correspond to the soul as it is understood in the Western context. Rather, it refers to a state, the state of the vital force of an individual. We can discern whether the *la* a person is weak from their physical and mental aspect, for instance, if a person looks totally distracted, is not aware, and physically looks a bit like a corpse. In this instance we say that their la is missing, and the truth is that the condition of the individual is very weak.

Nyen means ferocious, therefore *lanyen* means supremely ferocious. This is the characteristic of the illness. It can also be a singular disease of *lung, tripa*, or *peken*, or it can be a conjoined illness which already has a specific name. On top of this illness, there appears another illness caused by the invasion of another humor. But there is also a second scenario, in which an illness that has not been healed changes into another disease. These are called illnesses of transformation. There is a third scenario in which two strong illnesses are not conjoined, but in conflict with each other because of the clash of two humors. All these illnesses are usually called *lanyen*, and we think that they are always joined by provocations of an outside force.[8] Cancer, for example, which is very well known nowadays in the West, is a conjoined illness that manifests itself with this characteristic.

Western doctors interested in Tibetan medicine should understand a very important point, namely that the premise of Tibetan medicine, together with the concept of illness, is different from that of Western medicine. Actually, we do not have a precise correspondence in the translation of the terms we use; it is not easy to find it, because medicine develops also through culture, habits, and knowledge that are different in various countries

I will give you a simple example, not related to medicine, but still helpful to get a sense of what I am trying to say. When we go to buy meat, we can see that many butchers display a poster representing a

8   In Chögyal Namkhai Norbu's *Birth, Life, and Death*, Shang Shung Publications, Arcidosso, 2007, these illnesses are called "critical."

cow on which all the various cuts of meat are shown. In the Western world, there is a way to cut meat, and every cut has a specific name. Those who have this culture and knowledge will find it easy to translate those names from, for instance, English into French, or from French into Italian. But a different culture distant from the Western world, like the Tibetan or the Chinese, does not see things in the same way. So, if we translate the name of a very specific disease directly into Tibetan, it may not correspond, and this holds true also for cancer. We have this issue not only with cancer, but for any disease. Therefore, a doctor who really wants to understand Tibetan medicine must first of all study and learn the way Tibetans think and their way of seeing things. Based on my experience, I think this is very important. Even if I have read many books, I have found it difficult to understand Western medicine because many things do not correspond.

Thus, diseases that are difficult to heal in Tibetan are generically called *tren* (*skran*) or *dretren* (*'bras skran*): cancer fundamentally belongs to this category. But there are other kinds of diseases that are simply called *tren*. Another type is called *lhogpa* accompanied by *tren*, thus *lhogtren*. There are at least three principal considerations. As I explained earlier, cancer is not a single disease; it is rather a conjoined disease that is simultaneously in conflict with the contrast between two humors. This depends a great deal on how the disease manifests in an individual. Not all kinds of cancer are identical; each one has its own characteristic based on the individual.

In general, in Tibetan medicine we always hope to heal all illnesses and we try a way to overcome the problem at hand, but we do not always succeed. Many believe that Tibetan medicine can heal cancer, but this is not sure either. Tibetan medicine does not achieve miracles – people also have this fantasy a bit – but it does have important means. Even as far as pharmacology is concerned, as Doctor Jigme explained yesterday, Tibetan medicine is a natural medicine that utilizes a lot of substances like herbs, plants, fruits, minerals, precious minerals – in other words, remedies of all kinds. Through these remedies we have many systems of protection, especially against cancer: to prevent its formation, to block its development, to make it regress; and therefore it is possible to deal with it. At this level we use many medicines made from various ingredients, but we must understand that we are not dealing only with an organic illness (as we said, cancer has the characteristics of *lanyen* diseases), but that we must intervene on the function of the individual's energy. There is a type of cancer that we call *khonlhog* – *khon* means internal, *lhog* a kind of cancer – or *lhogtren* (the names are not important, if you do not know Tibetan they only create confusion), but it is a kind of cancer for which we do have a cure. At the beginning, we must slow its development and then eliminate it so that it will not have the strength to get worse. As a matter of fact, as you know very well, this kind of diseases spreads quickly. As we said, a type of cancer is called *dre* (*'bras*), and it is called this way because it is not just one organ that is sick, but on the organ or somewhere a nodule appears. At times on ill trees big knots appear: here the same thing happens. There is a way to block this development and once blocked to make it regress by intervening with medicines, but especially with mantras.

As I said yesterday, for a Western doctor it is really complicated to understand the use of mantras because a mantra seems a prayer, like turning to religion or to a belief. Of course, there must also be a belief at the root of the mantra, but I think that it is very important to really understand what it is and how it works. Mantra is a Sanskrit word, called *ngag* in Tibetan, which means formula. Usually these formulas are in Sanskrit because Tantra and its teachings originally came from India, but it is not always like that: there are mantras in many languages, even in languages we do not understand. Also at times mantras communicate a meaning, sometimes they do not. Does this mean that they have no meaning? Not really, most likely they had a meaning when these formulas were transmitted, when someone pronounced them, but we do not know the meaning or the language they are in. In this case, I am not talking about the Tantra teachings, because a mantra in Sanskrit surely has a meaning that we can study and learn.

Where do mantras come from? It is not always easy to state that they came from a saint, a bodhisattva, or a Buddha; it is not always like that. In general, in Tibetan we call a mantra *rig ngag* (*rig sngags*), whereas *drubpa* (*grub pa*) designates a person who has obtained this power, has pronounced these words. Why did they pronounce them? Because, as we said, the word is the fundamental symbol of the function of energy and is connected to voice, to breathing. Breathing is connected to the function of vital energy, of prana. If we want to make prana work and to coordinate it, one of the main means is breathing, which in turn is connected to the word, to sound. Then a fully realized being (for the Buddhist tradition it can be a bodhisattva, for instance) is full of compassion and wants to act on behalf of other beings. In which way? Since bodhisattvas have the capacity to work on the level of energy, they pronounce a secret formula putting the transmission of the function of energy in those words, in that sound, and let a person hear them. This is called the transmission of the sound of the mantra. After hearing it, people use it in their practice. There are mantras that must work through the three existences of the individual: body, speech, and mind. What does this mean? The instructions explain which position we must keep to practice and activate the mantra, and which mudra we must use (mudras are hand gestures). In certain practices, also a gesture has a specific power and function in communication. . The mantra can be recited under the breath so that we can hear its sound: this means that we have something to do with our voice to produce or realize this specific function of energy. Then we have many mudras that work also with mind. To overcome certain afflictions and diseases we visualize the garuda (a bird similar to an eagle) – a divinity very widespread both in the extremely ancient Bönpo tradition as well as in the Buddhist one. The garuda represents mostly the force of the fire element, which is a very powerful element able to elimi-nate or burn negativities. So, we use the visualization, or we can also say the transformation, of oneself in this form [i.e., that of the garuda], in this dimension. This corresponds to working with mind, and also the way to practice the mantra is mind's work. Thus, the mantra is presented with the three characteristics of our existence: as existence of form, physical body, and also as word. A formula can be spoken out or also written down; in the latter case, it is a concrete thing, written on paper.

There are diseases that according to the tradition of Tibetan medicine come from the class of beings called Tsa, a class believed to rule the force of planets. This force provokes the individual, disturbing their energy and causing the rise of various diseases usually considered very hard to cure, such as paralysis. In this case we have mantras that are simply printed and kept in contact with various parts of the body for a certain period of time. Officially mantras are not used that much in medicine because the doctor is mainly the person who makes diagnoses and prescribes medicine, but there are also therapies that require rituals and mantras conducted by specialists. There are also practicing physicians who are a kind of yogin who carry out this type of healing. In the end, all of this belongs to medicine because medicine is the science of healing, and if a disease cannot be cured through medications – which are the material aspect – we have the way to intervene on energy through mantras, breathing, and so on.

We also have the visualization of specific syllables on specific points in the body. Syllables represent sound. Let us take for example the letter A or B: when we read it, the first idea that comes to our mind is the sound A or B. And the sound itself represents force, energy. Thus, the letter, especially in the tradition of Tantra, is the most commonly used means to activate the function of energy. The written letter represents the form, the dimension of body; sound represents voice, energy; and concentration of visualization represents mind. This is a way to work with the existence of body, voice, and mind together – coordinating and activating the function of those aspects of our energy that are weak. This kind of therapy is always connected to the knowledge of the origin of diseases, of their actual condition, and of the means to cure them. An organic disease can be discovered easily with various analyses, but it is not always easy to discover if and when *dön*, provocations, are present as well.

There are specific analyses, for example of pulse and urine, to discover the presence of these disturbances, and all of them are connected to astrology. If we really want to discover the condition of the individual, their characteristics, their diseases, we need to examine their lives and their relative condition a bit. In this case the most utilized tool is astrology. In the West, these matters are not easily understood. For example, if a Tibetan has a complicated illness, they will go to a doctor that will conduct examinations and will discover the patient's illness is not only physical, but that there is also an energy provocation. If they are expert practitioners themselves, the doctor will try to discover the kind of provocation through astrology, or through various kinds of *mo* or divination. Astrology and *mo* are the fundamental means to discover things that cannot be understood in a direct fashion. For instance, to see a glass is direct contact: we can see it, touch it, we can understand it is a glass because we have direct contact with it. In the same way, examining a person we can have direct contact, and through analyses we can identify their disease. But we cannot discover energy provocation through direct contact: rather, to discover it we need to turn to an indirect method. For example, if we see smoke on top of a mountain, we deduct that there must be fire because we know that smoke comes from fire. In the case of medicine the method can be astrological calculations or *mo*.

What is *mo*? You prbaly have an idea of it because the book entitled *I Ching* is very well known in the West. *I Ching*, based on calculations of Chinese astrology, are useful to foresee many things when we do not know what to do or how to behave. In the traditions of ancient cultures there are many divination methods. For instance, I have seen in the West that people use tarot or read cards. At times people say that such readings are true, and at other times that they are not, and it is hard to understand if they actually work. Also, *mo* is a bit like that, although it seems like it works when the persons using it are practitioners with their own beliefs and knowledge of *mo*. In this kind of scenario, we do find an answer.

In Buddhist teachings and in Tantrism we think that practicing meditation is important. Why would this be the case? It is in order to develop clarity. If we develop clarity we can understand things better. *Mo* too has this function. In ancient times there existed, especially in Tibet, a very well known *mo* called *juthig* (*ju thig*). What is it? Practically speaking it consists of six strings that are tied in various ways and that create 360 main configurations from which, with small variations, more than one thousand different shapes can engender. The interpretation of each shape is often combined with astrology and explains exactly the characteristics of the individual and their circumstances. It is a rather interesting form of divination. Its interpretations were very much connected to the ancient uses and traditions of Tibet. Doctors used *mo* to discover specific illnesses hard to explain. They did not rely on it for all sicknesses, only for complex ones that could not be diagnosed normally.

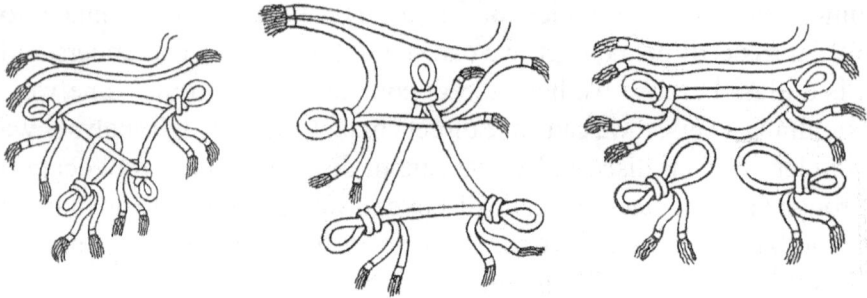

Figure 4. Example of juthig, from Chögyal Namkhai Norbu, Drung, Deu and Bon: Narrations, Symbolic Languages and the Bon Tradition on Ancient Tibet, Dharamsala: Library of Tibetan Works and Archives, 1995

There is also a simpler divination method called *deutrul* (*lde 'u 'phrul*) in which one uses forty-two pieces of crystal in various combinations. Otherwise we often do *mo* with the mala – a sort of rosary – or specific kind of dice. In tantrism divinations are not done randomly, but are instead conducted after specific practices whose function is to develop and realize clarity. We first do a little ritual and then the *mo*. So we obtain a result that at times is very useful and gives precise answers. As I have already mentioned, however, not all doctors do this and not for all illnesses, but only in the case of certain serious diseases like cancer. In this case we need first of all to diagnose the illness through very precise methods that deal with the physical body, like manual contact, pulse examination, observing diminishing appetite, mood changes, and so on. There are symptoms to analyze, but this is not enough; we need something more, and then we can be sure of the diagnosis. In Western medicine, it is not difficult to diagnose a tumor or cancer, but sometimes we discover it a bit late: this is the problem, and not only in Western medicine, but also in Tibetan medicine.

Based on my experience I believe that we have a slightly different way to perceive these kind of diseases compared to the Western viewpoint. I have noticed that here, when a patient has cancer, doctors decide to hide it from them and that they rarely notify the patient of the true nature of their disease so not to depress them. Of course, people need to be in good spirits to live well, and if a cancer patient becomes depressed, this already constitutes a problem. Thus, generally speaking, doctors prefer not to tell the truth. This can also happen in Tibetan practice, but there is also another way to perceive things. If the patient is a person who has understanding – meaning that they are able to collaborate with the doctor – and if it is possible to face and heal the problem through certain practices that work with the patient's energy, then in this situation we consider that we should not hide anything from the patient. It is better that they know – that they become aware and actively involved. If the patient has a deadly and hopeless sickness, there is no point in their knowing anything. But if there is hope that they can improve by collaborating with their doctor, knowing which illness affects them, they become aware and are willing to live and make an effort.

Therefore, I believe that we have two ways to see things that are slightly different in this regard. I am not talking about the different viewpoints in Western and Eastern medicine, rather about the question as to whether the patient is aware and collaborates with the doctor. There are people who cannot even comprehend what it means to collaborate and as soon as they learn that they have a serious disease like cancer, they immediately decide that there is nothing to do and that they can only die. Then it is not easy to convince them to collaborate. Often the disease is diagnosed too late, and even if someone is able to make miracles, it is not so easy. For instance, I meet a lot of people and maybe someone has heard that I am a Tibetan doctor, even if my work is not medicine, and they come to see me or call me and tell me that they have a serious illness. But in general, they always tell me at the very last moment. At times, it is the relatives that let me know about the illness, saying that their loved ones have been in therapy for years, but that now all doctors do not give them any hope of a cure any longer. And then they call me.

But what can *I* do? In this situation dealing with the problem is not easy even for Tibetan medicine. Many so-called incurable diseases, however, are not so in Tibetan medicine because the cure depends a great deal on the individual and on their condition.

When we know how the disease arose and how the patient's condition is, we have many ways to heal it, like medications or the use of mantras and many rituals. There are also therapies like moxa, for example, and many different kinds of needles. Many people ask if we have acupuncture in Tibetan medicine. Tibetan medicine has its own way to use acupuncture, but one of the most well-known and practiced cures in Tibetan medicine is moxa, while acupuncture is much more diffused in Chinese medicine. Many diseases caused by energy provocations are cured through moxa, which is considered a very efficient way to stop the development of diseases like cancer. We also use blood-letting, which also existed in the ancient tradition of Western medicine. When we speak about blood-letting you could think that that Tibetan medicine is a bit primitive. But we are not speaking just about letting blood. First of all, we must understand which type of blood is to be let and in which part of the body. What does blood-letting mean? We know that diseases, impurities, and toxins lie in the circulation of blood, especially in the case of liver diseases, and there is a medicine that can separate pure blood from impure blood. When we take it, the impure blood converges in the places from which we can let it out. In this way, we only remove the impure, sick blood, not the healthy one. When the impure blood is removed, so is the sickness. Afterwards we close the wound with moxa, a burn that blocks the disease and ensures that it will not come back.

There are many ways to use moxa. In Tibet, most doctors use the direct burn method because it is more effective, but there are also indirect manners that are very used in the Chinese tradition, for example using sticks to generate heat. There are four kinds of Tibetan moxa, and they are called *sowa* (*bsro ba*), *digpa* (*sdig pa*), *sepa* (*sreg pa*), and *tsowa* (*btso ba*). The first word means to heat. The second, dig, that we feel all the way to the bone: we do not burn the point directly, and it is very similar in worth to the Chinese tradition of acupuncture combined with moxa, which transfers the power of the heat. The third, *sepa*, means to burn, or to apply heat directly. The strongest kind is called *tso*, to cauterize, and it burns in depth. Some diseases must be burned this way, others not so very much. These means are very effective and can generally cure many diseases. But if there are energy provocations, moxa is considered one of the best ways to cure them.

Then we also have many rituals. For sure a doctor does not carry out rituals, but they can still recommend them as necessary because they know that to heal certain conditions there are particular methods. For Western doctors these are not easy things to comprehend, but it is not bad to have at least an idea about them, even if it does not mean we have to apply these methods. I would like to give an example that deals with a recent event – not an ancient tale.

I had an uncle who was a practitioner and passed away in 1960. He was not a doctor per se, but he knew how to heal many diseases because of his practice and his mantra capacity, which was very powerful. When I was a child, in my village people were often bitten by rabid dogs, and would go crazy and at times also die. So their relatives would bring these maddened people to see my uncle; I witnessed this many times.

Once, in particular, I saw two young people bring a man who was already delirious to see my uncle. He was bound, and at times he would bark or whimper like a dog. His eyes were red, and he was horrible to behold. He looked quite scary. They had brought him to my uncle because they knew that he had already healed similar cases. My uncle had that man sit in from of him and started reciting mantras. If the mad man had been able to recite the mantras himself, that would have been the best way to overcome the problem. There is also the possibility, however, for someone to intervene on behalf of a sick person, even if this concept is hard to understand. My uncle had a book of mantra practices (Tibetan books are long and narrow, and have a cover), and using that book as a stick he started to beat the mad man. The latter was quite strong, and even if the two young men were holding him tight, he kept trying to break free. I ran outside, and was afraid that the man would beat my uncle, but my uncle instead stood up and beat the man even more strongly. After a few blows, the man truly began to calm down, then sat down slowly and started to cry without putting up any resistance any longer. When I went back in I saw that the man was crying and trembling. They took him back home and the following day he could not move and was quite sick, but he was no longer crazy. He remained in that condition for four days: he was quite ill, very weak, but he could reason, and slowly he also started to walk. Finally, he got better. For Tibetans, this was not a miracle, as they are quite used to these things because many practitioners, and not only my uncle, do them. This story illustrates that the power of mantra exists concretely and can be of great help to sick people. But this principle is unknown in the Western world, especially as far as doctors are concerned.

This concludes my presentation, and my time is up, I hope I was clear enough.

Moderator for the day: Doctor Fernand Meyer

Doctor Lobsang will continue her presentation on gynecology and pregnancy.

LOBSANG DROLMA
Birth and post-delivery care. Breast cancer

Yesterday I spoke about pregnancy and the various stages of the growth of the fetus inside the uterus. This morning I will speak about the ninth month, the last one. Usually a child is born after about nine months and ten days, though we have cases where birth takes place in the eighth or even the seventh month of pregnancy. They say that if a woman rides horses, her pregnancy can last up to ten months. At the end of the nine months and ten days period, the child's consciousness begins to experience discomfort within the uterus and does not want to remain in it any more. The urgency to get out becomes quite strong. Just before birth, it is said that the child assumes the position in which they put the ring fingers in the respective nostrils. In the stage immediately before birth, the air energy called *dutse lung* moves the fetus in the right position for birth. The first signs of imminent delivery are, of course, the increasingly strong pains felt by the mother and the breaking of the waters that may happen before birth. After the breaking of the waters, before the complete dilation of the cervix that allows the child's head to crown, blood leaks. At that moment the child is in the position to exit the uterus headfirst. When the head is upside down and begins to emerge, the mother assumes the delivery position that, in the Tibetan tradition, is squatting, whereas in the West the position that is generally taken is lying down. In the former position, the face of the child comes out looking upwards so it is easy for the doctor, the nurse, or the obstetrician to remove all secretions from nose and mouth. If the child is too big, to ensure delivery the doctor's help is necessary, but the doctor must never force the exit of the child by child by pulling – helping delivery with gentle methods instead. In Tibet, we do not hold the child's head strongly nor do we pull it because this can cause cerebral damage. Furthermore, any strength applied to this area can later cause eyesight damage. Tibetan tradition prescribes making the child come out of the womb by delicately holding him or her with both hands to the sides of the head, above the ears.

In order to have a good psychological connection with the newborn baby, we believe that both parents must participate in the delivery. After birth, the mother pushes the extremity of the umbilical cord, and before tying a knot on it, she pulls it towards her in order to prevent any defect, deformation, and bad luck. This act is a gesture of good luck: she pulls it the first time to ensure the child will have a long and happy life, the second to ensure they will be free from illnesses, and the third so that they will have all kinds of capacities, well-being, prosperity, and a life without obstacles. The thread too is wound three times around the umbilical cord before tying a knot in it. This is an augural gesture to prevent diseases caused by conflicts between the three humors, *lung*, *tripa*, and *peken*. The cord is then spread out and cut about eight fingers from the mother's belly and four fingers from that of the baby. Cutting the cord less than four fingers can be dangerous for the baby because of all the movements he or she makes.

First of all, the newborn is washed, and then we put on their tongue a small pill with the Tibetan letter HRI as an augural symbol so that the child will develop great intelligence and wisdom and will be successful in their studies. HRI is the syllable of Chenrezig, Avalokiteshvara in Sanskrit, the bodhisattva of compassion, and pressing the pill on the baby's tongue as the first action creates a connection with the essential nature of the bodhisattva of compassion so that in the baby compassion, love, and kindness will spontaneously arise.

The second action is to spread a balm made with oil and butter around the belly button to prevent illness or local discomfort. The third action is to spread a medicine made of butter and herbs on the baby's soles because of the belief that it will develop perfect vision. It is true that thanks to the application of this medicine, almost all Tibetans have good eyesight without defects. The ingredients of these medicaments, for both mother and baby, are very simple, and I have a list here. We have now completed the topic of birth – describing a delivery with no problems.

Let us now turn to the complications that may arise in the last phase of pregnancy and during delivery, which are principally three. The first is when the mother loses too much blood. The second is when the mother eats too much and puts on too much weight: this hinders the birth due to the pressure of the mother's excess weight. The third may derive from the strength of the *lung* that, usually, causes the baby's head downwards, but that may push the head upwards, rendering the delivery process quite difficult.

During pregnancy, the doctor is able to establish if the baby is male, female, or if twins will be born. If the baby is male, the right side of the mother is higher; the baby's face is turned towards the mother's spine and this will cause her spine to jut out. Furthermore, her milk will first come out from her right breast, and she will feel light in her body and content in her mind. If the baby is female instead, the left side will be higher. The baby faces outwards and so the mother will tend to lean slightly forward. Once more there is symbolism in the position the two sexes assume *in utero*. Males have robust bodies, and the position of facing the mother's spine represents this strength, whereas females have a sweeter nature, and the forward-facing position symbolizes their gentleness. If the fetus is female, the mother perceives her body as heavy, her mind is somewhat uneasy, and has a general feeling of heaviness. She will also feel a natural attraction towards male company, and experience the desire to wear nice clothes and jewels. The doctor can also determine the sex of the child by taking the mother's pulse. Grabbing with strength the right wrist of the mother with the ring finger of the left hand, the doctor pushes until they feel the bone in order to take the liver's pulse. If the fetus is male, the pulse of the right kidney will be very strong. In the case of a female fetus, the opposite is true, that is, the doctor examines the mother's left wrist with the right hand's ring finger, and in the presence of a female fetus, the pulse of the left kidney will be very strong. In order to determine with certainty the sex of the fetus, taking the pulse only once is not enough; the doctor must take it many times, even up to one hundred times.

If the mother is pregnant with twins, her lower abdomen will stick out very clearly in the middle, and listening to it, the doctor will be able to hear two hearts beating. Furthermore, in general, if the mother is carrying only one baby, her complexion will darken slightly, but there are not many changes. In the case of twins, instead, her skin changes a great deal and becomes opaque; we see noticeable changes also in the mother's eyes, which become deep set, and in the cornea, which turns yellowish. The mother's face hair increases as well, and she can also experience leucorrhea. Urination frequency increases, and the uterus may prolapse. It is fundamental for the mother to see the doctor at least once a week because if the twins are not well separated *in utero*, we can have difficulties during their delivery.

Breast Cancer

We have completed the section on the process of pregnancy and delivery. We will now speak about the condition of the breasts. First of all, we will consider breast inflammations and infections. In a lactating mother, the breast at times can experience a small infection that can however develop complications and worsen. This is common among women who breastfeed but can also happen to women who are not. The first cause of infection that can manifest after delivery can be related to a lack of hygiene: the breast could be dirty or not clean enough. The second cause is a mother who is very busy that has no time to breast-feed the baby so that milk stagnates in the breasts causing tension. The third cause is the mother who forces her milk to dry up by stopping the breastfeeding of her baby. The fourth possible cause of breast infection is diet, especially if the mother eats too much mutton or drinks beer or alcoholic drinks excessively. The fifth cause are traumatic lesions due to accidents, falls, and so on. The sixth cause is the blockage or the compression of blood circulation around the nipples, for example due to wearing clothes that are too tight: blocking this circulation is very dangerous and can be one of the first causes of breast cancer. The breast increases in size and the skin turns very dark. It is very important to examine the breast to understand whether this is due to a tumor, and if so, to examine it to understand whether it is benign or malignant.

If it is a tumor, the woman may experience shivering even when she is in the sun or in bed. Internally she feels a stinging pain like if she were pricked with needles. As a matter of fact, if it is cancer, the white blood cells increase (we have red and white blood cells in the breasts) causing a sharp pain, like needle pricks, a very uncomfortable and almost unbearable feeling. This is the first stage of a breast tumor.

In the second stage, foul smelling pus develops within the breast that infects the skin and causes ulcers. In the third stage the lymphatic nodes under the armpits become affected, and they become hard and painful to the touch. It is not necessary for both armpits to become affected: if the tumor is in the left breast, the lymph nodes in the left armpit will be affected, and vice versa. If lymph nodes in both armpits are affected, this means that the tumor has spread, for example to the lungs or liver, and has done so through blood circulation causing metastases. This is the last stage.

I have used many special medicines of various kinds to treat cancer: some are very strong and must not be used in the first phase of treatment as they could cause problems. First of all, we must not use medications that are very strong at the start of treatment. We begin instead by giving medicines that will control local growth rather than a broad-spectrum medication, like an arrow that goes straight to the target. We give this first medicine to check the situation, and we monitor the reaction to it. After three days, the doctor checks its result and effects. The first medication is an infusion; the second is a slightly stronger powder; the third medication prescribed on the basis of increasing strength is a pill made with different herbs mixed together. After administering these three phases of treatment in sequence – the infusion, the powder, and the pills – it is possible to move on to the cure.

The last medication we administer is known as the "precious pill," a very powerful medication that we could compare to the atomic bomb that can destroy everything and that has many side effects all over the body. Thus, we administer it like the last resort when other medications have not given any results. If we use it at the beginning of the therapy, it can cause cell destruction and create many problems. It is very important to balance the medications on the basis of the patient's condition. For instance, to give a very powerful medication to an already weakened patient is very dangerous, while the same medication can be very effective for a patient that is in good shape. So the balance between the power of the medicine and the condition of the patient is fundamental.

Medications must be prescribed only after a careful and complete check-up and with full knowledge of all symptoms and health condition of the patient. It is important for the doctor to conduct a complete check-up, and to understand in depth the general make-up of the patient to calibrate and give the right medication at the right moment. After this last remedy known as the precious pill (rinchen), in the case of breast tumor we can use other treatments, such as moxa or moxibustion, in which we can use different kinds of needles. With the administration of this pill the tumor usually decreases in size, and so does the breast: this is the moment in which we can use gold moxibustion needles, positioning them all around the area in which the tumor was in order to eliminate it completely. If, after using the most powerful medication, the mass of the tumor remains extremely hard and wide-spread, we must use gold needles. If the tumor is not hard to the touch then we use silver needles. If after the various preceding stages, this last treatment is successful, the tumor will not return because it has been completely eradicated.

Breast cancer affects many women, it is the disease that most commonly strikes them. I will now talk briefly about some of the other most common diseases among women. The classification of the feminine conditions connected to this topic are, in order: menstruations; the conditions that arise during pregnancy; miscarriage and induced abortion; the conditions due to which a fetus dies *in utero*; hemorrhage during pregnancy; uterine prolapse; the conditions caused by residue that stay in the womb after delivery; eighth and last topic: poisons.

I will begin with menstrual problems, the majority of which affect women who have not given birth. The first problem is lack of regularity: sometimes the cycle lasts twenty days, or more, or less; usually it is irregular and during her period a woman feels great pain in her back, belly, or sides. There are many reasons why women experience these symptoms: first of all, tension and stress are factors that contribute to the emergence of menstrual issues. For instance, if a woman is anxious and worried about her job or other matters, this creates stress that will affect her cycle. Another reason could be the uterus being in an anomalous position, or a cervix that is too narrow. There could also be an internal inflammation or other issues inside the uterus, like tumors, fibroids, or cysts. An inflammation causes pain, whereas a tumor or a cyst do not cause painful symptoms. The first symptom of these conditions is a strong pain in the lower part of the abdomen, not a persistent but an intermittent one. The second symptom is an extended abdomen that swells and feels tense and hard. A third symptom is nervousness that manifests regardless of whether the woman is working or resting, and a tendency to be anxious and worried. Then there is vertigo, in this case persistent, and not intermittent. The woman can also experience unease in her heart region, in the central and higher part of her chest with clear swelling in her body, including in the legs and feet. The menstrual cycle becomes extremely irregular (it can take place more times in one month), with very little blood loss.

There are medications to treat this condition: first of all medicines, then diet, surgery, and life style or behavior. The reason we talk about life style is that a correct behavior makes the medicines more effective. The combination of medicines and life style is actually the best therapy. It is also very useful to trust the medication one is taking. A few patients get better after one day of treatment, others take their medications and benefit from them only after a long time. Thus, having confidence in the medications prescribed is important. This concludes the explanations on women's general conditions.

Questions and Answers

Question: What does Doctor Lobsang think and what does Tibet-an medicine have to say regarding therapeutic abortion or induced "criminal" abortion? Specifically, what is the future destiny of the fetus and what happens to the parents who want the abortion?

Answer: In Tibetan medicine there are many medications that can in-duce abortion, and the treatment is very simple. Tibetan doctors can induce abortion. However, they are Buddhists, and believe that taking a life goes against their faith, and so abortion is not practiced in Tibet. Based on Buddhist faith, inducing an abortion is a very negative action for those who carry it out. We can say that in their next life the parents of an aborted child will experience the fruit of their action which will definitely be negative. From the point of view of the baby, we can have two perspectives: the first is that in a previous life that baby had killed or caused somebody's death; the other is that in the future the baby, of course, will have to be reborn.

Question: What is the effect of the gold and silver needles in Tibetan medicine? In Chinese medicine the metal of which needles are made of is not important. What is their function? Thank you.

Answer: There are many reasons why gold needles are potentially considered very powerful and useful, especially in the treatment of cancer. Gold is an element that prolongs life and that has great power when it is used. It can influence cell growth, and so it is used especially in malignant pathologies.

Question: In which moment do you cut the umbilical cord?

Answer: We cut it as soon as the child is born and the rituals that take place after birth are completed, otherwise the baby will catch cold, which means that we cut it as soon as possible.

Question: Is there contraception in Tibetan medicine?

Answer: Yes, we do have contraception. It is well known, many people have become famous, especially in India, where it has been greatly advertised.

Question: Speaking of breast cancer, are needles put in specific sites on the tumor area, or are the points distant from one another?
Answer: We put the needles all around the tumor, about one finger-width one from the other.

Question: The doctor mentioned that breast cancer is one of the most widespread diseases among women. I would like to know why, and if this is only the case in the West, or also in India and Tibet. I would also like to know more about the contraceptives used in Tibet and if it is true that their effect varies in various climates
Answer: Cancer seems to be the most widespread disease in the West and in India, but it is rare in Tibet. The reason is the life style that Tibetans have maintained. The important thing in contraception is for the woman to be very precise in taking the medications. Climate has no influence whatsoever on their effects.

Moderator

Doctor Tenzin Chödrak was born in central Tibet in 1923. Between the age of ten and eighteen he took religious classes at Chode Monastery, and took monastic vows. He studied and practiced medicine at the Lhasa Tibetan Medical Center between the age of eighteen and thirty. In 1955, he became the personal doctor of the Dalai Lama, and in 1959 he was arrested and imprisoned until 1980. From 1976 until 1980 he practiced medicine in prison. In 1980, he was given permission to go to India, and currently he is the senior doctor for the Dalai Lama and the director of Tibetan Medicine Institute in Dharamsala, in Kangra District, Himachal Pradesh, India.

Tenzin Chödrak
Astrology and medicine

I am very happy to participate with all of you in this medical conference that has its goal to benefit others. Given that in this world all beings want to be happy and to avoid suffering, and that medicine aims to increase wellbeing and to free people from suffering, it is really great that you all are interested in this discipline, and thus I extend my greetings to each and every one of you. The presenters that spoke before me have already spoken about Tibetan medicine. Today I would like to briefly talk about the relationship between medicine and astrology. To treat this topic in a detailed way would require a lot of time and this is not the goal of this conference. We only introduce the topic in a way that will later allow for the development and the gradual deepening of knowledge. It is important to stimulate your interest so that these topics will become the door to further progress. So I will now give a brief introduction.

The corpus of Tibetan medicine is basically funded on four texts called the *Four Tantras*, or *Gyüzhi*. We are talking about more than six hundred pages, of which only three deal with the relationship between astrology and medicine. When we take the pulse of a healthy person free from disease, we can learn what will happen to them, to their relatives, if they are lucky, in good health; in other words, we can make predictions based on an astrological basis.

The seven examinations of the pulse

We have seven examinations of the pulse through which we can fore-tell whether we are going to be attacked by enemies, if something neg-ative is going to happen, if we are going to have a child, or how the father is doing based on the condition of the child, and so on and so forth. To take the pulse we use the index, the middle, and the ring fin-ger of each hand. With the index of the right hand we examine the fire element and the heart pulse. If the heart pulse is very strong, it will feel something like a swelling and rough. The right hand's middle finger is used to check the spleen pulse, which has a characteristic briefness. With the right hand's ring finger we can take the left kidney's pulse, whose element is water. This pulse is smooth and slow in winter. The left hand's index finger is used to examine metal, which is also the lung's pulse. The left hand's middle finger examines the wood element and reads the pulse of liver and gallbladder. The ring finger of the left hand reads the right kidney and also the bladder.

Pulse, seasons, and constellations in a healthy person

Let us turn now to the relationship between the pulse with constella-tions and seasons. As we said earlier, each person has a characteristic pulse that can be male, female, or neutral, that is, *potsa, motsa,* and *changchub semtsa.* This last one is also called "the pulse of the enlight-ened ones" or of beings that have a certain level of wisdom realization. But we are not going to dwell on this aspect, and we will focus instead on the relationship between pulse and seasons.

In springtime, because of the season's influence, most people will have the pulse characteristic of this season, meaning that the pulse that reads the liver and the gallbladder becomes quicker and thinner. In summertime, due to the seasonal influence alone, the heart pulse becomes automatically swollen and rough in most people. In winter the kidneys' pulse – whose element is water – is smooth and slow. If in summer, instead of the main fire pulse, that is, of the heart, we find the water pulse, that is, of the kidneys, which is slow and smooth, it is a sign that the person will encounter misfortune or setbacks. As we have already mentioned, we are looking at the influence of seasons – which means of constellations or astrology – in relationship to a healthy person. However due to the aforementioned condition, we can deduce that the person in question will encounter difficulties. This happens because fire is the natural enemy of water, and if instead of fire its enemy appears, we can predict misfortune. If instead of fire metal manifests – these two elements are not enemies, but friends – we can deduce that the condition of the person being examined will be good.

We have said that in the four seasons we have specific characteristics that influence the various pulses, and we are now taking summertime as an example. What happens when in summer we encounter a pulse that does not correspond to that of the season, which is the heart's pulse? We have already mentioned one, the pulse of the enemy, and we have said that it brings bad luck. Then we have examined the pulse of the friend, that of metal, which is a good omen. Then we have the pulse of the wood. Since wood is the mother of fire, if we encounter this pulse in summer, the mother-son relation foretells good things and a positive condition. We have examined the influence of seasons taking summer as an example. We can do the same with the other seasons. Examining the same relations of mother-son and enemy-friend we come to the respective conclusions. This is all about the topic of medicine in relation to astrology.

The three kinds of pulse

Let us now examine the three kinds of pulse, namely, masculine, feminine, and neutral. The relationship between these pulses in a couple determines their offspring and also tells us something of the characteristics of the couple. For instance, if both partners have a neutral pulse, the couple will not conceive. If both have a male pulse, the couple will have sons. If both have a feminine pulse, the children will be female. If, for example, the father has a male pulse – which is swollen and rough – and the mother a neutral pulse – which is smooth and slow – the couple will have only one or two children and then will not be able to procreate any longer.

Therefore, for a correct reading of the pulse in a healthy body in order to forecast the future, which diseases will arise and so on, we need to consider all these factors. The doctor must consider the masculine, feminine, and neutral pulse of the person under examination, as well as the season in which the exam is taking place while keeping in mind that, for each season, there is a specific characteristic element or one mostly influenced by the season itself. Taking in consideration all of these elements, the doctor can reach the correct conclusions, and on the basis of the signs or imbalances that the doctor detects in the pulse, they can predict the illnesses the healthy person will encounter.

For example, if in the summer months – during which the fire element is dominant – the pulse of the heart, instead of being swollen and rough, "sinks" and cannot be detected (we are talking about a healthy person), we can predict that the person under examination will be struck by paralysis, or will become lame, or dumb, or will lose control of some limb, or will have problems with their brain; or they will have foggy and obscured mind and will have to endure great suffering. If, instead, the fire pulse is swollen and rough in an excessive way we can foretell that the person will experience great fear and anxiety: perhaps because they will be attacked by enemies or damaged in various ways. And if that pulse has a special roughness, the doctor can predict that the person will have to face pain very difficult to overcome. If, in this period of the year [summer], the pulse presents a characteristic like that of boiling water, the doctor can deduce that the person being examined will have to endure a great deal of verbal abuse, unpleasant words, insults, accusations, and so on. If instead of the swollen and rough pulse typical of summer, we encounter the pulse of the liver, which corresponds to the wood element, since wood is the mother of fire, we can foretell that the relatives of the person in question (mother, aunt, uncle, and others), will encounter the above-mentioned problems with paralysis, and so on. The friend of fire is metal, and when we find the metal pulse subordinated to the fire pulse in this period of the year, all disturbances and misfortunes described earlier will strike the friends of the person being examined. Since water is fire's enemy, if we encounter the water pulse under that of fire in this period of the year, we can foretell that one's enemies will be struck by the misfortunes described above.

Pulses and Elements

We have taken as example summer and the dominant pulse in summer, the fire pulse, to explain the various relations we can have in terms of friend/enemy or mother/son, the way in which the various pulses that underlie the main pulse manifest, and the conditions that can be accordingly foretold. In the same way, each season of the year possesses a dominant pulse on the basis of which we can deduce the various possible combinations.

Another important factor is that seasons are the manifestation of the external elements earth, water, fire, and wood, which combine with one's own internal elements, and because of this interaction between external and internal elements it is possible to foretell what will come to pass. So, for instance, if we find ourselves in a place characterized by storms or strong winds, also our internal *lung* will react in relation to the manifestation of the external wind element. Or in summertime, when it is very hot, our fire element reacts to the external heat. What we have explained so far, as we have already said, always relates to a person in good health, with no illness. But through all these exams and the consideration of the relations between internal and external elements, between the seasons and all we have discussed up until now, we can predict an illness, a concern, or something else.

It is important for the doctor to carry out a preliminary preparation or preliminary exams related to the condition of the patient because the exam of the pulse can be influenced by various factors: as a matter of fact, what we learn from the pulse can be influenced by the behavioral habits of the patient. If, for instance, someone drinks a lot, or eats food that is too salty or too sweet, or if they never use salt, the pulse can be impacted, and if the doctor is not aware of these habits, they could reach the wrong conclusion by reading the pulse alone. For a correct reading of the pulse it is very important for the doctor to be very clear about all the aspects discussed until now, and to examine in depth the various characteristics connected to the seasons and the dominant pulses.

The pulse in a physically or mentally ill person

Let us now talk about someone who is sick just to emphasize the importance of examining the pulse correctly in order to exactly prescribe a treatment in relation to the symptoms. Some people, when they breathe, emit a loud sound that can be caused by an excess of bile, phlegm, or air: if we do not read the pulse exactly, the conclusion reached will automatically be wrong and the medications inappropriate. In this case the illness will not be overcome because in analyzing the pulse we did not pay enough attention to the conditions that correctly indicate the element in excess. Let us continue taking as an example a patient with trachea issues. In this situation, many factors can be at play. We could be dealing with a complex disease. The main cause of the respiratory issue could be phlegm, but on top of this, there could be bile or air, lung, problems. When more than one aspect is involved, and one of the three factors – bile, air, and phlegm – interferes with the others, the problem is doubled, and in order to be able to balance the humors and to heal the disease we need to prescribe medications that heal different aspects. If we heal only one of the factors and we do not consider the other, the disease will not be cured.

Let us now turn to another disease, namely, diabetes. In Tibetan medicine, there are ten kinds of diabetes that we can divide into three groups on the basis of the urine, which can be clear, whitish, or with sediments. From these three basic groups, the combinations derive: some kinds of diabetes show complications coming from heat, like fever, others coming from cold, and so on, for a total of ten. As far as high pressure goes, for instance, in Tibetan medicine there are four pathologies in which hypertension can be present: we can encounter it in a weakened body; in a patient who drinks too much or eats too much meat; or it can be due to lung. The doctor must be an expert, and carry out a careful examination because only a correct diagnosis allows them to prescribe the correct medication.

In the case of a kidney disease, if there is fever, medication is called for, but the lack of an accurate diagnosis will cause further problems because various kidney diseases depend also on the habits of the patient. For example, drinking too many sweetened drinks or eating too many sweets damages the kidneys. So the doctor needs to be aware of each different aspect, otherwise they can prescribe the wrong medication. Let us take the case of another disease, for instance, a stomach dysfunction. Some people cannot digest very well and believe that this is due to a lack of heat in the stomach. So they go to the doctor's and say: "I do not have enough heat in my stomach, I cannot digest well, please examine me." But when the doctor examines the patient with care, they find that there is heat in the stomach, and that the digestion is difficult because the three elements air, phlegm, and bile are not balanced and create problems. This is the cause of indigestion, not the lack of heat. If the doctor is not experienced or does not carry out an in-depth visit, they could be influenced by what the patient says. But the patient can be wrong because they do not have great knowledge. Therefore, it is very important for the doctor to conduct an in-depth and complete examination based on their own knowledge and experience.

As far as cancer is concerned, we have treated patients with cancer of the kidney, stomach, intestine, colon, breast, tongue, or nose. After a correct diagnosis we were able to prepare medications, and some patients got better, and others did not. I will stress again the importance of an in-depth check-up and of a correct diagnosis: only in this way can the cancer be discovered, perfectly individuated, and treated with the right medication.

These are a few examples of illnesses that affect the body. Let us talk now about mental illness. Basically mental illness is ignorance, that is, the ignorance of not knowing one's basic nature. Because of this ignorance, the three emotions, attachment, anger or aggression, and stupidity arise. On this base the three humors, air, bile, and phlegm arise. When we speak of physical illness, we speak of a disease caused directly by the three humors. But the manifestation of an illness has deeper causes that have to be found in the mind: the basic ignorance of mind is the source of all the diseases that manifest in the body. The three passions are the immediate cause of organic diseases, but everything can be traced back to ignorance – the original cause.

Other components of the body, aside from the three humors, are the seven essentials, namely chyle, blood, flesh, fat, bones, spinal fluid, and reproductive fluids (sperm and eggs). There are also the five elements. Only if these three factors – the three humors, the seven essentials, and the five elements – work correctly together and are balanced, the body is healthy and can develop and work properly like it is in the case of the family, which can prosper only if all its members work together towards a common goal. In this way, good fortune increases and the common effort moves towards the right direction. If this does not happen because family members start arguing and begin to compete to decide who is stronger than the others and so on, then disharmony reigns and there is no hope to reach the common goal. The same holds true for the body: only if the fifteen components work together as one, in the right balance, body and mind are healthy and everything works appropriately. But if this does not happen, all kinds of illnesses arise. Basically, things cannot be harmonized, because, for example, water and fire are opposite elements. What we mean by working in balance is that each of the various factors works at its own level as a whole, in a general balance, without one being dominant and another being weak.

Moderator

I would like to add a few words to clarify that astrology and medicine are not restricted to what Amchi Chödrak, due to time constraints, spoke about. Actually, in medical texts we find divination through pulse taking, like Amchi Chödrak explained, and also through urine analysis: but this is only one kind of astrology that Tibetan doctors are used to deploying. There is also a more traditional form of Tibetan astrology more connected to constellations, seasons, day of birth, the events connected to the moment of birth, and it is a science usually taught to doctors. As a matter of fact, the Men Tsee Khang, the University of Medicine in Dharamsala is a university of medicine and astrology. And there is a very important part of astrology that is not taught in medical texts but in particular texts strictly related [to it]. Therefore, astrological medicine is not restricted to pulse and urine. Thank you.

TSARONG JIGME
Pharmacology and pharmocodynamics

Ladies and Gentlemen, I will first of all present briefly on pharmacology. Afterwards, since I believe that it is important for you to see what we do concretely, we will show you some slides of the ingredients we use, and Doctor Chödrak will explain their properties, their specific usage, and so on. If you recall the introduction I gave the other day, the basis of pharmacology is, of course, matter, which is based on the five proto-elements Earth, Water, Fire, Air, and Space. This is the key to understand all of pharmacology. The combination of Earth and Water engenders *peken*. As an aside, I believe we have to use the term as is because its translation can cause confusion, since *peken* has nothing to do with phlegm. So, I prefer to use the original word, explaining, if need be, what it means. I believe this is the right approach, even if others may disagree. Then Fire engenders *tripa*, and air *lung*.

Let us talk now of their properties or intrinsic qualities. What are they? For instance, Earth is heavy (*chiwa*), stable (*tempa*), tender (*dulwa*), and from these properties an individual can receive certain qualities like kindness, and so on. It is fat, and it is also dry, *kampa*; it also has the quality to amalgamate and it pacifies or controls *lung*. Water is *lawa*, humid, liquid, and *silwa*, refreshing, and it has weight. And so on and so forth.

The Six Tastes

The Six Tastes derive from the proto-elements. The combination of Earth and Water engenders the sweet taste. We are also talking about the post-digestion taste: we eat something, we digest it, and the taste changes. After the digestion, the sweet taste remains sweet. The combination of Earth and Fire engenders the sour taste, and after digestion, the taste remains sour. The combination of water and fire produces the salty taste (*lentsawa, lan tshva ba*); after digestion, the taste becomes sweet. Water and Air produce the bitter taste (*khawa, kha ba*); after digestion, the taste remains bitter. Fire and Air produce the taste that some call pungent (*tsawa, tsha ba*), but I think that pungent is more about the smell, which is spicy. Spicy food burns the mouth, like red peppers and pepper. Earth and Air give the astringent taste, and after digestion the taste becomes bitter.

Now let us go back to the proto-elements. Earth pacifies or controls *lung*; Water pacifies *tripa*; Fire *peken*; Air pacifies both *peken* and *tripa*; and Space is pervasive.

I do not believe that it is important to discuss the Ayurvedic system: we find six tastes also there, but we explain them in different ways, and in Ayurveda they also use Space which for us is omni-pervasive. Let us now see the effect of taste on the three processes. The sweet engenders *peken*, but controls lung and *tripa*. The sour engenders *tripa* and pacifies *lung* and *peken*. The salty engenders *tripa* and pacifies *lung* and *peken*. The bitter produces *lung* and *peken* and pacifies *tripa*. There is a very bitter salad that is very good for the liver, and thus this is the principle, as the bitter controls bile in excess. The spicy produces *tripa* and pacifies *lung* and *peken*. The astringent produces *lung* and *peken* and pacifies *tripa*.

The Pharmacodynamics of the Six Tastes

Let us now enter into the pharmacodynamics of the Six Tastes. Sweet food, if eaten in moderation, is very nutritious, is good for the body, increases the seven constituents, enlarges the corporeal mass, is a tonic for the elderly, children, and the weak, soothes the throat, clams coughing, helps wounds heal, eliminates toxins, purifies the five senses, and pacifies *lung* and *tripa*. If eaten in excess, it causes weight gain, reduces body heat, imbalances *peken*, causes obesity, polyuria, and acne. Excess in salty food causes hair loss, premature grey hair, wrinkles, weight loss, increase in thirst, skin diseases, and imbalances *tripa*. Taken in moderation it dissolves any physical block, induces perspiration, especially through hot compresses, develops body heat, and increases appetite. If taken in moderation, bitter food increases one's appetite, calms one's thirst, is antibacterial and antitoxic, and cures fainting, infections, and *tripa*; it dries fat, oil, marrow, urine, and feces. Taken in excess, it weakens the seven constituents, and imbalances *lung* and *peken*. Spicy food eaten in moderation provides heat to the stomach, acts as a digestive, increases one's appetite, heals throat illnesses and dries fat and infected tissues. In excess it decreases sperm production, weakens the body, causes tremors, fainting, abdominal and lumbar pain, and dries fat, blood, and infected tissues. Sour food taken in moderation, develops body heat, increases the appetite, calms one's thirst, controls diarrhea, acts as a digestive, develops the sense of touch, and opens channels blocked by lung. If in excess, it imbalances *tripa*, increases indolence, weakens one's sight, makes one thirsty, and lowers one's immune defenses, making the body more prone to infections usually accompanied by nausea. Astringent food, if taken in moderation, heals wounds and increases the luminosity of one's complexion. In excess it imbalances *peken*, it leads to bloating, blocks the body's channels, increases constipation, and causes a general weakening of the body and heat disturbances.

Pharmacological ingredients

Now the most important or popular *materia medica* is the *Shelgong sheltreng* (*bdud rtsi sman gyi rnam dbye nus ming rgyas par bshad pa shel gong shel phreng zhes bya ba*) written by Geshe Tenzin Phunt-sog in 1717. This manuscript lists 2,294 main medical substances, of which we find various kinds, up to even five different ones. So, it is a very large corpus. The other day I mentioned the various materials we use, like the *rinpoche* or precious medical stones, rocks, animal prod-ucts, and so on, therefore it is not necessary for me to go back to this topic. With these medical substances we produce various medications like *thang* or decoctions, *rilbu* or pills, *chema* (*phye ma*) or powders, *degu* (*lde gu*) or medical barley soups, *menmar* (*sman mar*) or medic-inal butters mostly used as ointments. There is a famous *menmar* for *lung*, made with, I believe, nutmeg mixed with butter used to massage the hands and the soles of the feet that are very sensitive body parts. There is then an ingredient known as *talmen* (*thal sman*) which means medicinal ash. It means that you take a metal, for example, and you oxidize it and pulverize it using a pestle and mortar. Then there is an ingredient called *khanda* (*khaṇḍa*) which is decoction, but is made by letting it boil on a very low flame, filtering it, and then boiling it again until it becomes as dense as syrup. Then we have *menchang* (*sman chang*) that is a distillation made from various medicines, it is a *chang*; then we have *rinpoche*, and finally *ngojor* (*sngo sbyor*) or mixes of plants and medical herbs. Now we will show you the slides and some of the ingredients we use.

SLIDE 1 This is the Medicine Buddha, I thought it would be appropriate to show him to you. You can see that he holds a plant in his hand, and this the way in which you can recognize the Medicine Buddha. It is interesting because we do not have very ancient statues of the Medicine Buddha. There are some conjectures about the origins of this particular statue, with some people saying that it could have been made in Afghanistan.

SLIDE2 This is a statue of Yuthog Yönten Gönpo the Elder. He holds in his hand a medical plant known as *aru namgyal*, which is a bulb of the same species of the *terminalia chebula*. There are different kinds of arura, and this is the *nampar gyalwa*, which is unique. He is also holding a manuscript found in the original Pali Sutra teachings by the Buddha, the Tengyur. This manuscript tells of the Seven Medicine Buddhas, each of whom made a vow to always help the sick who think of and meditate on them, on their energy, and so on.

SLIDE 3 This is a depiction of the Five Elements. This is Wood, in the form of a deity. This is Fire, and then Earth, Space, and Water.

SLIDE 4 Here is an example of some of the spices we use, known as *sangpo drug* (*bzang po drug*), the six auspicious substances. Doctor Chödrak can explain them more in detail.

Doctor Chödrak:

The six auspicious substances are nutmeg (*dzati 'dza ti*), beneficial to the heart; bamboo pith (*chugang, cu gang*), beneficial to the lungs. Its real ingredient comes from bamboo, it is a secretion from it, but you cannot find it any longer, everything is synthetic and there are problems with this medicine. Then we have saffron (*kurgum, gur gum*), beneficial to the liver; cloves (*li shi*), beneficial to the central channel; and *kakola, (ka ko la)* a kind of cardamom good for the stomach and the spleen. The green cardamom *sugmel* (*sug mel*) is ideal for the kidneys, and benefits also all the six vital organs. We put a small quantity of each ingredient in medicines because the idea is to balance their actions so that their respective side effects will not damage the other organs. Each has its own specific action.

Doctor Jigme:

SLIDE 5 This is another example of a medical formula, and again you see many plants. I will not deal with the details of the recipe, it is only to give you an idea. These untreated materials will be dried, cleaned, weighed on the basis of a specific recipe and finely ground, and are ingested as powder or pills.

We now see a series of minerals and precious materials, and I will turn to Doctor Chödrak to explain their properties and functions.

Doctor Chödrak:

Mumen (*mu men*) is effective against poison and disturbances of fluids, lymph, and leprosy. We never use it by itself, but always in mixtures.

Coral (*byi ru*) is helpful to lower blood pressure. All these ingredients are used in mixtures, and never by themselves, so we do not take some coral saying, "bye-bye, high blood pressure!" We must boil these substances and detox them, and so on. I am showing you some of our ingredients to give you an idea.

Turquoise (*g.yu*) helps the liver and works as an antidote against poisons, always in mixtures. If you take it by itself, it will heal the liver, but damage the stomach and the intestine, and so we can use it as the main ingredient but also mixed with many other medical substances.

Gold (*gser*) is effective against aging, preserves the dewiness and the luminosity of one's skin and is effective against various poisons, mostly alimentary ones.

Trago (*khra mgo*) is a shell we call hawk's head. It helps bones and nerves. How to use it? First of all, we need to purify it by boiling it – so it is written in some manuscripts –   then we mix it with various medicines. Otherwise one's stomach's heat will be damaged, or even eliminated, with serious threat to one's life. We also deploy other methods to purify poisons like iron rust, oxidized copper, and so on.

Kandi is found at great heights, and is a variety of chalk helpful especially in illnesses of cold and hot nature, or inflammations of the liver, and of liver *lung*.

Do thel (*rdo thel*) is used to get rid of stomach tumors and against indigestion. Even in this case it is the main ingredient, but it is not very effective when used by itself. We have to use it combined with other ingredients.

Do in *do le* (*rdo klad*) means pebble, *le* means brain, because it is shaped like brains, and has a wonderful smell. It is helpful to treat the brain. I do not know the geological term.

Sulphur (*mu zi*) is used mostly for lymph matters. I repeat, all these minerals need to be detoxed, purified, and pulverized, and there is a whole procedure to it that we must follow.

Calcite or *chong zhi* (cong zhi) is used for *peken* (phlegm) and gastric ulcers.

Stalactites and stalagmites are varieties of calcite, and they contain calcium. In this slide you can see the untreated material, and in the next one you can see the detoxed final product that will eventually be pulverized.

Venice, April 29, 1983
Morning (first session)

Moderator for the day: Professor Barrie Simmons

BARRIE SIMMONS
Psychotherapy, self-acceptance, and tibetan medicine

Given my role as moderator for today's presentations, and as the first presenter, I will introduce myself. My name is Barrie Simmons, I am American, but I will speak in Italian, given our location, and as I am under the perhaps mistaken impression that the majority of people here are either Italians or understand this language. I am a psychotherapist and a student of Buddhist teachings, especially Tibetan ones. This morning I will talk about psychotherapy, Tibetan medicine, and self-acceptance, as this last topic is, in my view, one that brings together these two forms of practical knowledge. I imagine you are here for two main reasons. You are interested in the topics of this conference because you want to learn something useful for your job, be it medicine, education, or any other discipline aimed at helping others. You are driven by the desire to discover new possibilities that will make what you do even more effective, but I am sure that many of you are interested in change for your own lives as well and that you expect, as a result of these days' experience, something that will help you directly.

Therefore, I encourage you to clearly keep in mind these two goals as you listen to the very little I will say and to the important words the others will speak after me. I take for granted, because of my professional bias, that everyone entering this room, will have brought with them two minds, namely, the conscious mind that listens and tries to understand, reasons, estimates, comparing its convictions and logic with what is being said here, and the unconscious mind, which is listening in this very moment independently from the conscious mind. The unconscious mind is always listening – always interested in capturing any stimuli, symbol, meaning, experience that may be enriching, and useful for the growth and personal development I mentioned earlier. At times the conscious mind triumphs; at times it falls short of the situation. It would have already helped us had it been able to do so. Today I am trying to speak to the conscious mind, though I am aware that in any event I am also speaking to that incredible wealth and depth that is in each of us and that psychology, with its poverty in language, calls unconscious

The three themes, psychotherapy, self-acceptance, and Tibetan medicine, I want to discuss today could in some sense be considered three ways to talk about the same thing. As you know from having listened to the speakers who presented their work in these days, Tibetan medicine is rooted in the vision that we call Buddhist in the West, but that for Buddhists and Tibetans is simply the vision of *how things are*, and the doctrine of *what is there*. In the Buddhist analysis of *what is there*, of *how things are* we can roughly say that the answer to the question of *what is happening* is *nothing*. But things keep happening. There is a basic emptiness, a continuation of events, happenings, that is the dimension in which we find ourselves, and there is also *how* it happens – the way in which what is happening takes place and is described as energy. To put it even more bluntly, from this perspective matter is like *distracted* energy that does not know how to recognize and understand itself, whereas matter would be energy that is *integrated* and totally self-aware.

Already in the foundation of this vision we thus have a discourse of awareness – a recognition of what one person is and of [what it means] to live in one's own dimension. Things are the way they are, and yet they are not fully what they are until they become aware of it. They are not fully their existence until they recognize what that existence is. We could perhaps say that in this sense body, speech ¬ word, or energy, as we heard – and mind each are a little closer to becoming aware, or to being able to become aware, than what they are. We could also say that when the body is not just what it is, but becomes aware of what it is, we have what is called realization – the full recognition also of the material dimension.

Tibetan medicine originates from this fundamental vision (and we have here a methodological choice) which, as we shall see, is very important, because being relative and not absolute deals with provisional things and does not simply apply the application of the fundamental vision we have heard called "dharma." Of course, medicine works with what is there, but it deals with provisional, temporary things, and so it deals with corporeal problems mostly through physical means; it deals with problems and disturbances of energy mostly with means that relate to energy, which in other words affects breathing and sound – means that deploy energy to intervene on energy. Finally, medicine deals with mental problems by using means that are connected to mind. We have a difference here – which is actually not a real difference but simply a matter of emphasis – between medicine and teaching, and it is the fundamental vision behind medicine, that of course works with full recognition of the existence of body and energy, but also aims towards working directly with mind in order to then bring the results of an awakened perception to bear upon all the areas of an individual's existence.

Psychotherapy belongs to the history of the West and was born in a specific historical moment less than one hundred years ago and developed historically in many ways, at certain junctures in a way that was not fully aware of its own self. It developed in the West, however, when people increasingly realized that neither society nor institutions could heal individual persons and their personal problems, and that this task fell to the individuals themselves. Was this due perhaps to a moment of historical crisis, in which society and institutions were less convincing to the individual, or perhaps to a juncture of growth, in which the individual living in the West began to discover themselves as less dependent and noticed how they themselves were the protagonists of their own existences? I do not know which one is the right answer, and I do not even know if we are dealing with two different things or only one phenomenon.

In any case, psychotherapy is born at a very specific historical moment with the project to heal the individual, in one sense, from themselves: a cure of the mind with the means of the mind but also, at least in modern psychotherapy, a healing, through the mind, of other dimensions that we can call here body and energy. With this project, psychotherapy distances itself from historical and institutional Western psychiatry – which tries instead to work on mind, energy, on the individual through external interventions or the administering of material substances – and posits, even if often in an unclear way, the resolution of personal problems through the re-awakening of self- consciousness through what we can call awareness.

Psychotherapy quickly discovered that the self is not an object, a thing, that there is nothing *there* other than a series of events, a process, a becoming. The self is thus defined, at most, as the *place* – meant as a space defined by what happens within it, but empty in and of itself – where a certain type of process, of development, is happening. Psychotherapy works with the idea that each of us has a self-image, in a way an idea of how things work, and believes that this idea is something objective. For psychotherapy, at least in the way I understand it, this idea of the self, this self-image, can to a large extent be true because it is deduced from real experiences – I have observed myself in specific situations, and I have understood what I am like – but it is also the product of how *they have told me what I am like*. In any event, it is just an idea, i.e., a fantasy.

Plato already taught us that ideas are eternal, perfect, geometric, symmetrical, clear, whereas reality is confusing, contradictory, changeable, alive. Even the contrast between self-image and the reality of the process of continually becoming, but empty in and of itself, which constitutes each of us, has these characteristics. The idea of who one is, one's self-image from a psychological view, the models one swallowed, the roles one learned, the rules one obeyed, the expectations of others one tries to meet, all of this, therefore, can sooner or later clash with the changeable and contradictory reality perceived by the person one is. These two things are not without relationship and connections, but at a certain point in one's existence there can be a full conflict between the person one imagines oneself to be and that which one truly is.

Psychotherapy aims to address this suffering by making the individual face their existence and experience, leading them not only to understand but also to experiment, feel, and live all those dimensions – impulses, desires, memories, feelings, experiences, capacities, shortcomings – that make up their reality but not the image they have of their own selves. These dimensions exist, but they are not acceptable by the conscious mind I mentioned earlier or are so only in theory. I have an image of myself in part because I have understood who I am in specific circumstances that by now are no longer the reality in which I am living, in part because I have committed to believing myself to be in a certain way because at a certain moment of my existence this choice aided my survival. And later, in order to maintain this idea of myself, I am forced to reject most of the reality of what I live, feel, perceive,and experience. I do not want to face a great part of my experience and learning; I do not want to be aware of it; I throw it away in the treasure chest, underground, or the universe that psychologists call unconsciousness.

How come individuals adhere to the idea they have of themselves so intensely that they deprive themselves of their own existence, to the point that they give up the richness of the reality that could be – and is? The psychotherapist would answer that individuals, finding themselves living in a dimension one could call freedom or emptiness (and this could be due to historical factors or attributed to the fundamental nature of existence), must face a situation in which there are no clear guidelines while life keeps asking them to judge – choose, no matter at what cost – and to endlessly take responsibility. So, they adhere to a certain self-image in order to have a road-map, to have an external reassurance after all – a self-image that is external as individuals are not yet themselves, their own existence, their own awareness. If we can no longer depend on God, demons, magic, science or religion, we can still depend on our own self-image, a construct that is external to ourselves and in which we mirror ourselves instead of diving in the reality of our experience and choices.

Psychotherapy tries to promote the contact between individuals and their direct experiences, the realization that arises from the experience of what is, of how it is; the acknowledgement of one's own responsibility when one realizes what one is doing and that therefore they can also not do it or choose to keep doing it, with the awareness that one is living one's existence and not being lived by external factors, as it were, and that even when one is lived by external factors, also this is one's own choice.

Let us turn now from psychotherapy to self-acceptance. We do not need to change image or metaphor. Psychotherapy aims to the acceptance of the self in a radical sense: to live oneself, to be aware of oneself, and to take responsibility for oneself are not three different things, but three different ways of saying the same thing. What is self-acceptance? It is not only understanding oneself, which would only be a division between the one who understands and the one who is understood. It is not only approving of oneself, where we find the same division between the one who approves and the one who is approved as well as, on top of this, a constant search for one's own approval, as tortuous and challenging as the search for others' acceptance that leads to the sort of self-torture that is self-improvement. It is not resignation, which is far from being self-acceptance and is instead the most radical of disqualifications: I am worth nothing and there is nothing to do about it.

Self-acceptance consists of experiencing oneself physically, emotionally, intellectually, in any given moment without the inhibition of self-assessment, self-judgement, self-criticism; to be in oneself two – one who looks and manipulates the other. This being there and being one with oneself is not enough, one needs to be aware of it: one is not who one is if one does not know it. And it is very difficult. It is not spontaneity, but full presence. To be what one is, to being with what one is, intellectually, emotionally, and physically, goes against all of our habits. "How am I doing? Am I doing OK now? What are they thinking of me now? Am I doing the right thing? Am I close to my own ideal of myself?" These are our thoughts in each moment, our methods to manipulate and alienate ourselves.

We are talking here of a project that is the very opposite of all of this autohypnosis, of all this self-conditioning, of all that self-manipulation that is our habitual condition. When one is, or gets close to be what one is, when we move past the pleasure and the advantages of not being there, we discover astounding things, such as, for example, in psychotherapy a concept of normality quite different from the one many of us are accustomed to. In psychotherapy, a normal person is someone with great and painful inner conflicts, with strong and painful external frustrations, who is aware of and is in touch with these conflicts and frustrations.

In psychotherapy, the normal individual is not someone without inner conflicts and external frustrations. This condition, from a psychotherapeutic point of view, defines a corpse, not a living person. Then the difference between normality and abnormality, between sickness and health, is not the presence or absence of conflict, the presence or absence of frustrations and challenges, but the presence or the absence of awareness and contact with oneself. From this perspective, if it is normal to have conflicts, to solve them by making certain choices means to experience the birth of new conflicts. If the constant [cycle of] polarization/solution/repolarization is normal for the individual, then normality becomes being who one is and not approximating some model, some external normative construct. Then the rejection of the reality of who one is, is not fear, but fear of fear; not anger, but anger directed towards oneself and towards a world made of anger; not horror, but horror of horror. It is not conflict, but conflict with oneself about having conflicts. That is the illness, that is, the attempt to obfuscate, deny, escape the situation in which we truly find ourselves. The health psychotherapy aims for is therefore not the abolishment of the so-called negative, but the acceptance of the phenomenon of human beings, of the phenomenon itself as is.

Psychotherapy, after the birth of the psychotherapeutic dimension of psychosomatics, takes in consideration also physical illness – the illness of the body. From the psychotherapeutic perspective, the fundamental characteristics of physical illness are retraceable to either conflict with one's self or with the external world, and in the absence of awareness about said conflict, absence of realization of it, of identification with what one is. To put it roughly and simply, also because we are short on time, and due to my own limitations as a speaker, this vision presupposes that one can experience conflict in their own mind and be aware of said conflict, or that one can store it in one of the other pockets at one's disposal which are only two, namely, energy – that which at times psychologists call behavior, movement, sound, word, or, if you wish, unconscious – and body. There is no fourth pocket, no other place in which to put the conflict. If I choose not to be aware of a certain conflict, or if I do not manifest it because I cannot, or if I bury it in a way that is a bit dangerous for the body, that conflict ends up coming out anyway: it does not come out as it is, but it comes out nonetheless. At the physical level, we call a symptom this meeting between something that wants to express itself and its inhibition. It may begin as a tic, an itch, as the tiniest unease, to eventually become a symptom, to grow and become an illness, and, eventually, a funeral. Bringing back the conflict to the level of awareness, to the level of mind, is one of the projects that psychotherapy shares with the vision of the teaching behind Tibetan medicine.

In summary, today I suggested that what brings together psychotherapy, Tibetan medicine, as well as the vision and the teachings behind it, is the project to awaken oneself from what one is not and to accept and become what one is.

Venice, April 29, 1983
Morning (second session)

Moderator

Now we shall have the honor and pleasure to hear Professor Rakra Tethong Rinpoche speak about teaching in a Swiss community.

PROFESSOR RAKRA TETHONG RINPOCHE
The education of Tibetan children in Switzerland

Ladies and gentlemen, I am here today only as a sign of respect for Professor Namkhai Norbu who organized this great conference about Tibetan medicine. I was not planning to speak and did not prepare any speech, but Professor Norbu asked me to speak, so I am obliged to do it because we have been friends for a quarter of a century. For the past twenty-three years I have taught Tibetan children at the Children's Village Pestalozzi, in Switzerland. Of course, we heal children because education is a cure, a kind of cure of the mind that for me is the spiritual part of medicine.

I do not have much to say, but I would like to speak a bit about Bön and Shang Shung from an historical point. Then I will speak about the Five Elements, and finally, of course, I will speak about the job I do in Switzerland.

Bön and Bönpos are very important for the development of Tibetan medicine as well as for the history of Tibet. Tibetans today find themselves in the position of having to re-discover their Bön origins. Whether they like it or not, the time has come to do so. I am not speaking about the religious aspects of Bön, but of the results of my readings in history, ancient testimonials, and texts written in Tibet's ancestral language and orthography.

Bön, and the land we call Böd – i.e., Tibet – are terms we use nowadays, but in the past words were different. In the ancient texts, we do not find the word "Bön," but rather "Ön," or sometimes "Pön," with the "p" pronounced strongly. This term did not refer to a king or to a single individual lineage; rather, it indicated in general a person of great quality, culture, and capacity. Or we can see in the ancient texts that Böd – Tibet's present appellation – indicated the country, and Bön, its people. In the countries bordering India and Nepal and all the way down to India, local languages referred to Tibet with words like Bot, Botya, Botha, and so on. In ancient Sanskrit, the most common word for Tibet is Botata Himalaya. In the local dialects of the regions of Kalimpong, Darjeeling, or Kashmir, they refer to Tibetans with Botya even nowadays.

We cannot reach a definitive conclusion on the term with which Tibetans were called thousands of years ago, but we can reckon that this sound may have something to do with the original name for the region. "Bhutan" is a corruption of the Sanskrit word "Bhota," i.e., Tibet, and "anta," border, meaning the region bordering Tibet. But it has been a long time, many generations already, since Tibetans have ignored Bön from the point of view of literature, history, and science, considering it instead only in philosophical and religious terms. Bönpos themselves nowadays are interested almost exclusively in their rituals, religious practices, and customs, and are not aware of the history that preceded them. We can say that this is true in general for all Bönpos.

In any event, in the history of Tibetan Buddhism for the past 1,200 years there has been a fertile exchange between Bön and Buddhism: Bönpos conformed to Buddhism, and Buddhists adopted Bön elements. For instance, in Buddhist rituals we use drums and cymbals that are ancient Bön instruments: music from the double-sided hand-held drums and cymbals is not originally Buddhist. The swastika was, in origin, a Bönpo symbol. Today Buddhists in Tibet and all Tibetans see the swastika as an auspicious symbol because they think that it has an intrinsic value, stable and unchangeable. When a lama conducts a ritual on someone's behalf, or when we officiate a wedding, or start the construction of a new building, we believe drawing a swastika is important. The Bönpos have a long lineage of rituals and mantras, and for this reason people believe that Bönpos are basically shamans. But not all Tibetans believe that Bön is basically distinct from Tibet's other religious traditions. For instance, the great yogi Drukpa Kunleg stated that the white tradition of Bön is identical, in its essence, to the Buddhist tradition. And the famous lama Khangsar Dorje, when he visited Lhoka, examined some Bön texts and concluded that the Bön tradition was identical to the Buddhist philosophy Yogacara/Cittamatra. Consequently, people who do not know a tradition can nurture wrong prejudices. The horror of some Tibetans towards Bön, similar to the horror of many Westerners when they behold a swastika, comes from a failed understanding. This is what I had to say about the Bön tradition, and I will now turn to the topic of Shang Shung.

Shang Shung is a particular region that is an extremely important source from which Tibetan science developed. Shang Shung was originally called Kinar or Kinnara. In Tibetan, we call it *miam ci* (*mi 'am ci*) that, more or less, means "humanoid" or "humanoid vehicle." The reason why the term Kinnara was lost and replaced with Shang Shung is due to a king of the Shang Shung lineage and to his hegemony over the entire region. At any rate, the historical documents of Shang Shung dealing with the epoch of Songtsen Gampo (seventh century) are very clear. I cannot prove that Shang Shung underwent an enormous development in ancient times, but we can see that it is adjacent to north-western India, and that it had exchanges and relationships with that part of India as well as with Afghanistan, Kashmir, and so on. And already back then religious practitioners from those areas went on retreat in the Himalayas, and in order to get there they crossed Shang Shung.

Due to the challenges to preserve them locally, the old traditions and sciences of ancient India were brought to the Himalayan region. As far as location is concerned, Shang Shung is a region in India, beyond the city of Shimla, called by Tibetans today Kinnaur, or Khunu. Why do I claim that Kinnaur is the original territory of Shang Shung? I got this idea from an extremely great teacher, Khunu Lama Tendzin Gyaltsen. But why am I interested in these things and involved in them? Many, many years ago, my ancestors came from Kinnaur, and until three or four centuries ago the location of Shang Shung was known, and people called that area Shang Shung. We have sources that allow us to make this claim. For example, we speak of a famous poet who lived five hundred years ago and wrote in Tibetan. His name was Shang Shungpa Yungwa Tragpa, and Shang Shungpa indicated his place of origin and had therefore to be a common appellation.

I will now speak now of the Five Elements about which, in these past few days, many doctors have already spoken. As you must have noticed, they often mentioned metal and wood. According to Buddhist customs, we speak of the elements of earth, water, air, fire, and space; metal and wood, as elements, derive from astrology. The Five Elements are tightly connected to the five mental poisons, which are attachment, anger, ignorance, pride, and jealousy. These poisons are not external; they are something subjective, inside of us, and when their essence changes, or, in other words, when they are transformed, they become the Five Wisdoms.[9] There is a close relation between the five poisons and the five elements. For instance, fire, or heat, is the condition that gives rise to the negative emotion of desire; desire is characterized by heat. When heat, or fire, is transformed, discriminating wisdom arises. There is therefore a tight connection between the five physical elements, the five negative metal emotions, and their transformation into the five wisdoms.

Now I would like to say something on my career. I arrived in Switzerland in August of 1960 with my wife and small son because the Kinderdorf Pestalozzi, the International Children Village, had decided to welcome twenty Tibetan child refugees. At the time, I was working in the All-India Radio Tibetan Unit in Poona, and the government in exile asked me to take a few child refugees, so I brought twenty-one of them to the Kinderdorf Pestalozzi. That first group was made up of Tibetan refugees. We still had many problems with India, so, at our request, the village offered us a second house that we inaugurated in 1965. As of today, we have housed eighty Tibetan children. My work with the first group, as well as with the second one, is done, and I am now working with a third group. My main task is to teach children our

---

9   The Five Wisdoms are: the wisdom of dharmadhātu, the mirror-like wisdom, the wisdom of equality, the discriminating wisdom, and the all-accomplishing wisdom.

language, history, grammar, and some basic religious instructions. This is what I have been doing for the past twenty-five years.

It was not easy to launch the work in this international children's village. I had to learn how to teach Tibetan language, dance, and music in a way appropriate for children. Luckily, I love dance and music, including Indian and Western classical music, very much, and so it was not so hard for me to teach. Now the work with the first cohort is over, and they all have jobs, families of their own, and they live in good conditions and many already have children as well. Between one task and another, our youth meet for conferences and cultural events because many among them love to learn more about our religion, our traditions, our literature, and so on.

In Tibet, in the last centuries, Tibetans seriously studied philosophy and religion, learning logic and medicine, but all these activities were under the hegemony of the monasteries. Commoners had no access to this knowledge and were only schooled in a very general way. And I believe that this was a big mistake: for many centuries Tibetans did not go beyond elementary education, and thus there was a big gap between religious and lay culture. Common people, even if they take a few courses, find it very difficult to understand the religion and philosophy of their own country, and this is becoming increasingly clear. Now the time has come for the Tibetan youth to gain access to our religion, literature, and culture. Even His Holiness the Dalai Lama believes that we have to teach more about our culture to our youth and children, and offer them more opportunities to study.

I have talked a lot about this with my friends. Many say that it is important to create a bridge to spread our extremely rich Tibetan culture: of course, it is important, but it is not easy. Our ancient culture is like an opulent castle on top of a high and solid rock, but the head of the bridge on the other side, in which our youngsters and normal people live, is fragile. Their knowledge is like a sand hill, we cannot build on top of it. I do not want to stop hoping, however, and I think that, instead of a bridge, it is best to build a ladder. Perhaps, with a ladder, the children can slowly, slowly, ascend. But when we think of children, when we think of the poor Tibetan children, waiting for them at the top of the ladder is not an easy task for myself and other scholars: we must descend and help them raise their cultural level.

My formal training took place in the Drepung monastery. I was a monk until 1929, and I went to Gyumed, the renowned Tantric monastery, where I completed my studies. I love Sanskrit, I studied it for six years at the University of Calcutta, and then I was an assistant researcher in Poona for three years. I have studied all of our rich literature, but for children it is important to learn a simple Buddhist literature – fairy tales, stories, we have a lot of them. Now it is the time to make things a bit simpler, and this is why I teach. And if someone were to ask me: "What will you do in the future?" I could easily answer that I will write children's books. This is my plan. Thank you very much, and my thanks to the translators

Moderator

Thanks, Rakra Rinpoche. Doctor Tazan would like to say a few words. Doctor Tashi Tazan, a Tibetan by birth, has a degree in Western medicine.

DOCTOR TASHI TAZAN
The Tibetan Youth Association in Europe

Ladies and gentlemen, greetings. I wanted to speak in Tibetan, but since there are not many Tibetans in the audience, I will speak in German. It is very important, and it is a stimulus for the young Tibetans who live in Europe to see that many people in the West are interested in our culture. I think that this deep interest is a concrete proof of the fact that Tibetan culture is indispensable for humanity. I will speak to you about the Tibetan Youth Association in Europe. Many Westerners have asked our Tibetan elders if also the young Tibetans who live in Switzerland or Europe are interested in keeping Tibetan culture alive. I believe that many of you have asked themselves the same question, or will do so in the future, and therefore I think that it is useful to try and give you an answer.

As Rakra Rinpoche said, from the beginning of the 1960's many Tibetan groups arrived in Europe because many Westerners took the destiny of Tibetan people to heart, and some even offered material help. We have Tibetans in Germany, Great Britain, France, and there are various settlements also in the German-speaking part of Switzerland. The first time the Tibetans living in all of Europe could meet was on the occasion of the laying of the first stone of the Tibetan Monastic Institute of Rikon. Young people met elders, and they exchanged ideas and came up with the idea to meet more often to create a group to meet our needs, to exchange views, and to teach our culture to others.

In 1970 a small group of young Tibetans, in collaboration with the representatives of His Holiness the Dalai Lama, invited all the other young Tibetans to go to Rikon, close to Winterthur. A lot of them came, and we spent three days together on the shores of Lake Zurich. The topic we discussed was to find ways to transmit Tibetan culture to our youngsters in order to preserve its integrity also in Europe. The consensus was to create an association, and so, in 1970, the Tibetan Youth Association in Europe (TYAE) was born, with its seat in Zurich. Its main goal is to first of all create connections among all the Tibetans in Europe, and then to protect Tibetan culture in Europe, to help financially all the poor Tibetans in India, Bhutan, and Nepal, and finally to organize public interest events on the problems of Tibetan people in India and elsewhere.

The association is managed by board of eight members and is divided into seven interest groups, each of which is headed by a person. These groups are called sections. One section deals with Tibetan music: we play, we perform in events organized by the Association, and anyone who wants to learn how to play a Tibetan instrument can do so. Another section, Chölsum, deals with the organization of events and Tibetan holidays. Other sections organize trips, spring excursions, summer holidays, camping trips, and so on. Every year our festivities, including the celebration for His Holiness the Dalai Lama, are a great attraction and an opportunity for the 1,400 Tibetans living in Switzerland to meet and participate in the event. We also organize events with Swiss people, because we believe that it is essential to let them know about our culture and to include them in our activities, creating friendly connections and promoting peaceful coexistence. During the summer holidays, when there are many events in touristic destinations, we organize kitchens and stands where we sell food and Tibetan specialties, and with the earnings we support financially thirty-three children in Dharamsala, providing for their elementary education.

We help first and foremost Tibetan children in India. When we got to Europe, His Holiness the Dalai Lama told us – and we remember this very well – that the future of Tibetan people is in the hands of the young. These words were etched in our minds, and through our work and our association, we have tried to make them become real. Therefore, we aim to help and sponsor the primary education of Tibetan children, but we are still not able to make Tibetan culture accessible to our European friends in their own languages, because our linguistic knowledge is not yet up to the task. We hope that, by promoting education among the young, we will be able to improve the information and the communication between East and West, and that this will be mutually beneficial.

Our organization also organizes meetings between the various sections because we believe that Tibetan culture is not learned only through books. We know that certain things can be learned only from books, but one cannot become a Buddhist only by reading books; one must learn the rituals, the culture, one must speak Tibetan, at least a little bit. We believe that Tibetan culture can be learned only in contact with Tibetan people – living it in the first person – and for this reason it is very important to organize events and festivities with the Tibetan elders. An average of eight hundred to one thousand people take part in these events, and young people can then bring home with them shared experiences and memories that they can then transmit to others. If you wish to have more information or to support our job, get in touch with us.

Another goal of our organization is to make our most secret wishes come true. Tibetans want to go back to their country and we hope that, as time goes by, things will change so that Tibetans will no longer be forced to live abroad as refugees and that they will be able to return to their land. And in order to do so, we need your help. Thank you.

NAMKHAI NORBU
Medicine and Yantra Yoga

I will now speak about Yantra Yoga. One could say: "What is the place of Yantra Yoga in a medical conference?" What is known as 'yoga' in general and yantra yoga in particular – together with teachings on meditation, healing rituals, and the function of mantras we discussed yesterday – does not properly belong to medicine, but still is connected to it because, like we explained, the individual is made up by body, speech, and mind. If we want then to overcome an illness or a physical ailment, we must be aware [of this fact]. From this perspective, yoga becomes a very important tool, especially to resolve energy problems and disturbances.

Let us begin first of all by analyzing the word "yoga." These days yoga is quite widespread in the Western world – Hatha Yoga particularly so – and is often translated as "union." It is true that the Sanskrit word has this meaning. In Tibetan, however, yoga is translated with the term *naljor*, which does not mean union. *Nal* means one's nature, one's natural condition as is, just like in Tibetan medicine the three humors *lung*, *tripa* and *peken* – terms by now we have become familiar with – that are not a disease in medicine but one's natural condition. When our humors remain unaltered in their condition, we are not ill. Therefore, *nal* indicates the situation in which a person's conditions of body, speech, and mind are in their perfect nature. *Jor* means having this knowledge, this condition. So, we do not always use "yoga" to mean "union."

To begin with, people often ask whether yoga is a religion or a sport. [In order to answer this question] we need to get a better sense of what "religion" means. In the West this word is used often and is easily understood as the relationship between god and human beings. On this basis, representatives of different religions, and not just Christianity, but also Buddhism and Hinduism, who want to collaborate – I myself have been invited to many interreligious meetings – do so by searching for a God, because they believe that religion is about the relationship between human beings and God. So, they gather and together they go and search for God. But there are other ways to understand things [when it comes to religion].

For example, in Buddhist teaching we do not speak of religion but of "Dharma." Dharma does not indicate the relationship between human beings and god, but the true condition of existence. It is a different way of seeing things, a different way of thinking. How do Buddhists see Christianity then? They understand it as the Christian way of understanding existence. If they have explanations regarding God, this is a point of view; but the term Buddhists use is existence, the condition of existence. As you can see, "religion," or Dharma for Buddhists, is based on the knowledge and the cultural heritage of an individual and of various countries. The other day we talked a good deal about Bön, the ancient Tibetan religion. Bön means "to recite," because its followers believed that reciting mantras and conducting rituals was very important. It is not a way of understanding existence like Buddhism, rather one recites mantras and works at the level of energy to make energy work in a certain fashion. Bön was a blanket term to refer to all the religions of the time and not just one. The same holds true for Buddhists: Dharma does not refer to one specific religion – Buddhism – it refers instead to existence as a whole.

Therefore, it is not easy to decide whether yoga is a religion, even if in the end what we mean with the word "religion" deals principally with the communication of a specific form of knowledge. Also in

Buddhism we have different schools, and different institutions, but these differences are relative to the teachings that became integrated over time with the culture of a specific nation. Clearly this is not what Buddha taught, since Buddha transmitted knowledge.

The same holds true for the teaching of yoga. For instance, we can ponder the differences between Hatha Yoga and the practices of exercise and breathing called yantra in the Buddhist tradition. There are not great differences when it comes to the movements and breathing per se, what is different is the *way* of utilizing them. The true difference lies in the fact that Hinduism and Buddhism are tied to different philosophies and points of view. And what is the philosophy? It is what in Buddhism is called "existence," the existence of a human being. It is not enough to speak of body, speech, and mind because we consider that body, speech, and mind have their own essential nature. In Buddhism, we speak of nature of mind because mind is more important than body and energy.

For us the body, the material dimension, is easier to understand, because we can touch and see the body. In modern society changes, revolutions – which, according to some, are carried out for progress's sake – in countries and societies happen at the material level. Everybody speaks of economic problems, such as, for example, [world] hunger. Hunger arises from material things, so people struggle to solve the material issues connected with our material body, to our material dimension. This is what "body" means, not just our physical body, but also the all the matter that surrounds human beings.

Aside from the body, we have speech or energy, which is more challenging to understand because we cannot see or touch it. But we can communicate it, for example with words and sounds. In the Tantric Buddhist teachings, we often use the term *dang* that specifically refers to the condition of sound, to the capacity of sound to communicate. Many songs are called *dang* because through songs one can communicate, just like with mantras. Thus speech – which is the same level of sound, which is in turn the same level of mantra – is something more complex and harder to discover than the material body. We do have, however, ways to understand it and communicate it.

Mind is even more complex [to understand] than voice because we cannot hear it with our ears. Mind reasons, and thoughts continually arise. When we think something negative we are disturbed by it and other problems arise. All of this is not considered the state of existence, which is instead the fact this complex mind has its own nature, its own condition. This is often explained through the example of the mirror that helps to understand the condition of the individual. Glasses are meant to see an object, but a mirror helps us to see ourselves. With the help of a mirror one sees oneself, the condition of one's existence, namely, material body, energy, and mind. These three aspects – that we call the relative condition of the existence of the individual – have their own state, their own condition or nature. Even if we can confirm nothing, thoughts arise continuously just like reflections in a mirror. If we put an object in front of a mirror, the mirror will reflect it, and in the same manner in the mind thoughts of all kinds arise, good and bad, and through the function of the energy of such thoughts actions arise, and through actions one can develop physical problems.

Where does all this originate? It arises in the mirror that symbolizes the nature of mind. What is the nature of the mirror? And we are not speaking just of the matter by which it is constituted, but also of its potential to reflect anything that appears in front of it, be it a positive or a negative object. When we speak of meditation, we mean a method to enter the condition of one's own state. What happens when we find ourselves in our true state? We can understand this again through the example of the mirror. It makes no difference to the mirror whether it reflects a pleasant or unpleasant object, but beauty and lack thereof affect those outside the mirror who judge its reflections, i.e., those who take these reflections to be real. This is the way in which acceptance or rejection arise, and this is the principle that is usually called dualism, whence our attachment originates.

Many people do not give importance to attachment, but it is a crucial factor in all problems in our lives. For instance, if a child swears or insults an adult, the latter will not get upset with a child who, the adult will believe, does not understand what he or she is actually saying. At most the adult will think the child is rude and will leave it at that. If a professor, a doctor, or a person deemed to be important, however, uses the very same insults, this person will feel nervous and very much offended. Where is the difference? Is it in the words perhaps? No, because we have already stated that the child and the professor use the very same words. The difference lies in the person on the receiving end of the insults and the weight they give to these words. This is what we call attachment, and it is the source of our problems. This is the reason why we must understand our own state, or nature of mind, which is like the condition of the mirror. The mirror does not enjoy or dislike what it reflects, regardless of whether it is pleasing or unpleasant. But this happens only when one is aware and finds oneself in that state.

Nal, nature, means this condition, and in this condition all possibilities exist, just like reflections in a mirror. A mirror that does not reflect is no longer a mirror: this is the way in which it displays its capacity. Thus, reflecting images is not a defect of the mirror – that is not where the problem originates. The problem comes from not understanding one's condition and from being outside the mirror. That is where dualism comes from.

It is not enough to understand this point through words because words are dry and lifeless: it is necessary to understand a little in a practical fashion. This means that we need to understand our condition. In our condition, there are aspects that concern the body, and there is energy, and finally there is mind. If one does not know this, a lot of knowledge can become a fantasy. For instance, someone can read a book about yoga or Buddhist philosophy and say: "How very beautiful, how interesting!" But this person does not become realized, nothing changes for him or her. We need to have a concrete experience: things become interesting when we apply knowledge. To do so it is not enough to know theory, we need to know how to do it in a concrete way. So, we need to understand mind depends on energy, and energy on the body, and therefore we need to work with the body as well.

Let us take the case of a boy or a girl who is not happy. A lot of young people find themselves in situations in which they do not have a good relationship with their parents, or in which they feel lonely, even if they have siblings and friends. Day after day they shut others off and their situation worsens. One can encourage them perhaps to remain open to others, to keep calm, and not get agitated. Everybody is good at giving advice, especially parents, but these are not effective words, as they can actually make these young people even more nervous because nobody likes to feel nervous and alone. How come they cannot relax? In order to do so it is not enough to think that one does not want to feel nervous because underneath it all, it is the energy function that does not allow it. But we do not understand this. At times, we get this wonderful idea: "Today I have nothing to do and I do not have to go to work. I want to take it easy." And so, we get ready to drink a cup of tea and maybe read a book, but in reality we continue to be agitated, and we never relax. There is a Tibetan proverb that says: "Pigeons spend the entire night getting ready for bed." And indeed, pigeons keep turning, now left now right, to find the most comfortable position from dusk until dawn.

This happens because we do not understand that the function of energy does not allow us to relax. It is important to grasp this point, and if we do not understand that energy exists we cannot realize the ideas of the mind. But energy also depends on the material body: its function is connected to breathing and to the various movements of the body. For instance, inhaling while seated is different from inhaling while standing, and holding one's breath while twisting one's torso is different from doing so while sitting straight. Movement and position, in other words, are important. In yoga, we often use this saying: "Mind is like a lame horseman, and prana like a blind person," meaning that horse and horseman can travel far if they collaborate, but that each, on its own, gets in trouble and is not very efficient. Therefore, yoga and similar practices become a very important means to reach concrete knowledge, and they are not simply like reading a book.

We can cure a disease in four fundamental ways: diet, behavior, medicine, and various therapies. Behavior is also connected to practices like Yantra Yoga. In the West, Yantra Yoga, unlike Hatha Yoga, is not very diffused. These two appear similar, but in Tibet Tantra has different schools and traditions. In turn, each of these has its own practices to concretely reach knowledge through body, energy, and mind, and to be able to enter in the knowledge of the nature of mind. It has its own practices in which positions and movements are used that are called yantra. Yantra is a Sanskrit word very used also in Hinduism, and it indicates forms, many forms. The Tibetan equivalent of this word is *trulkhor*, which indicates not only the form or position, but also the movement. The principle of Yantra Yoga is therefore quite different from Hatha Yoga, in which position is very important: in Yantra Yoga movement is more important. At the same time this does not mean that there are no positions in Yantra Yoga.

There are many Yantra Yoga traditions but the one I would like to explain, because I know it personally and have experience of it, is Yantra Yoga that was introduced by a seventh century Tibetan teacher called Vairochana. He wrote and transmitted a text, which includes a special way to practice yantra in which each position is connected to one of the seven kinds of breathing. In Yantra Yoga breathing and movement are connected, and this is very important. We also have preliminary movements that are fundamental to learn how to breathe. It seems a bit funny to say this because everyone breathes. And it is true, everyone breathes, but this does not mean that everyone breathes naturally because, as we said, breathing depends on the mind. You can see this very well when you observe someone who is very agitated and breathes in a way that differs from that of someone in a calm state. Also, someone who is asleep and is having a horrible dream will breathe in a strange way, and at times they will also jump and scream. This means that there is no breathing that is really natural because we are conditioned by mind. Therefore, it is important to learn to breathe in a correct way.

This too is not easy. We have become accustomed since childhood to breathe in the way in which mind responds. Our parents – and especially our grandparents – love us, address us with terms of endearment, take us in their arms and cuddle, but they do not teach us to breathe well; they do not pay attention to this issue. But even if they did, it would not be an easy task. And not only parents, but also institutions do not care about teaching us how to breathe. Parents think that schools fix everything, but unfortunately schools do not teach you how to breathe. This means that unfortunately we ignore the condition of the existence of energy. The only discipline that explains and applies breathing is yoga.

Unfortunately, at times yoga encounters many obstacles and resistance because people are limited and reject it simply because it belongs to an Eastern culture, or because they think it is a religion and they have another faith, or because they are lay, "scientific," modern people. The problem, in the end, is not so much to accept yoga or not, but rather that people do not understand their own existence and do not know how to utilize things. Learning yoga does not mean to apply a position like a Buddha statue, or to show that one follows an Eastern teacher, or to wear an Eastern dress, or to make some strange scene: the principle is not this. The fundamental point is to understand one's own existence and to do one's best to use the means one has.

In Yantra Yoga we have first of all movements to coordinate breathing. But even this is not simple: if we were dealing with a visible object, it would be simpler because we could show it and explain, but breathing is an internal matter, connected to the function of energy, and we do not know what is happening or how things are going within us. For this reason, in general the different types of yoga should be learned from an expert teacher, and this not in order to create a bureaucracy, a tradition, or a school, but to guarantee a correct learning of breathing. Breathing is not something we see: we can explain how to breathe in a certain way, we can read a manual, but at times it is not easy to understand what is happening, and this is why we need an experienced teacher.

Therefore, in the preliminaries of Yantra there are movements that are very important to guarantee correct breathing. Then the teacher teaches the principle to guide the prana, energy, and its characteristics. Everybody knows how to breathe in and out, but there are many ways to do it: there is the direct way, indirect way, holding, and there is also the method to guide the breath in different parts of the body. Why do we need to learn these breathing methods? If we want to minimally stabilize in a practical way the knowledge of breathing, we need to train and apply these methods, otherwise we will not be able to change the habit of breathing in a disorderly fashion, which is what we have from birth. And we do not solve the problem only with one or two days of correct practice. By applying effective methods like the various holds, however, we can balance our breathing and obtain results in a relatively short time. Many people in the West believe that to hold one's breath for a long time is a show of skill; others even think that it is helpful to remain under water for a long time. Of course, if one is able to, there is nothing wrong with it, and one can use this skill, but this is not the principle. The principle is rather to establish a correct way to breathe in our daily life.

The practice of Yantra Yoga must not be understood as a medicine that we take for a couple of days to heal a certain illness; this is not the principle. The principle is that we need it to stabilize energy so that we can continue to live with a certain rhythm and in health. If we have prana disturbances, Yantra Yoga also helps to coordinate prana, to make it work anew. In order for this to happen concretely it is not enough to work only with breath: since we have three aspects in our existence – body, speech, and mind – we need to work with all three jointly. Using certain bodily positions we control breathing, and when breathing is controlled, so is the function of vital energy. All of this is guided by mind. In yoga breathing is very important, but it is not only breathing that controls prana: prana is especially guided by mind, and this is why we need to use visualization or concentration.

You may have seen various yoga books where we can find drawings of the human figure with the central and lateral channels, along with many chakras, which are the points where the channels meet and from which the vital energy moves to the various parts of the body. Thus, there are precise points in our body we need to visualize. With visualization, together with breathing and holds, we concentrate prana, the vital energy, in a specific area. In Yantra Yoga we also have the therapy aspect, but this does not mean that yoga can replace medical therapies. Since an illness is always related to energy, however, in yoga teachings we explain that illness is first of all a manifestation of a prana disorder.

For instance, madness manifests because prana enters into certain heart and lung channels in which it should not circulate. This means that in various parts of the body we have the function of prana – which is not exactly breathing – and that guiding that vital energy with mind we can coordinate and activate it.

I will give you an example related to therapy within yoga. If a person has a problem with their knee or foot, which are points far away from the abdomen, how can they guide the prana through breathing? We hold our breath, at most we can hold it at the level of the diaphragm, and the breath does not get to the foot. But through visualizing that point in the body, together with breathing and the control of the body through a certain pose, we can guide the prana. Of course, the benefit will not come in one day.

At times, Western people have strange ideas. Once, when I was at the university, a professor asked me if it was true that telepathy existed, meaning the ability to transmit or understand someone else's thoughts. I answered that it was possible because this phenomenon is related to clarity, and if an individual's clarity is developed, also telepathy is possible. The professor agreed with me, and added that he had tried to do it at few times, without any success. I answered that trying two or three times it was going to be very difficult to succeed: there are practitioners who retreat to the mountains for years and still fail to engage in telepathy easily.

So, many people think that if they have pain in their knee they just need to concentrate and the pain will go away, but it is not really like that. In yoga, like in many other things, one needs to train. One needs to train breathing – controlling also one's pose. Once one becomes more familiar with these practices, if one really knows how to guide one's breathing and understands certain techniques, yoga does work. Knowing how to unite body, speech, and mind is extremely important. We can easily understand this with one example: if we want to light a fire, we need matches. But taking a match in one's hand is not enough to produce fire, we need a matchbox or something to strike the match against. And even this is not enough, as we still need someone to strike the match. When we have all this, fire manifests, it works, it becomes real. Just so, understanding first of all the three aspects of existence and knowing how to use them all at once, we have the possibility to manifest something concretely.

If you are really interested to practice Yantra Yoga, you must first of all learn precise movements aimed at achieving correct breathing. This is extremely important. I know many people who are a bit interested in yoga: they go to the bookstore, buy a book, and begin to make certain movements and breathings. Sometimes this can be fine, but it can also be dangerous: we can play with many things, but not with *prana*. For example, in the book we just bought it may be explained that holding the breath – called *kumbhaka* in yoga – restores youth, prolongs life, or gives one certain powers. And this way some people become fascinated by this idea and every day they lock themselves in their rooms, fill their bellies with air, pull up and down, and eventually end up with a sickness in their bellies.

Nowadays there are also many people who buy books on *kundalini* practice – very diffused in the West. I am not saying that if they understand the instructions well and know how to do it this practice will not bring benefit: *kundalini* energy is a power that can bring many benefits. But perhaps they breathe in a certain way that forces too much, and then things can go bad. This means playing with energy. It is better to play with the physical body: playing with a ball, or, even better, swimming, are very beneficial to health. In yoga, we must not play with *prana*. We need to learn from an expert teacher, one who knows how to teach and can guarantee a perfect breathing. Learning how to breathe perfectly is a guarantee of a healthy life.

But we need also to understand that there is something more, that breathing is not enough to balance body, speech, and mind. We must not forget what the base of the condition of an individual is. In Buddhism in general the base consists of the two truths: relative and absolute. What is absolute truth? It is not something mysterious: it is the nature of mind – its true condition that is like the condition of the mirror: clear, pure, and limpid. An individual who understands this and tries to be in this condition in a stable way becomes free from all problems, whereas if they only do physical exercise and breathe they only manage to have good health.

For example, if we put a pot of water on the stove, when the water starts to boil, it begins to come out of the pot. We can then add a bit of cold water, so that the water cools down, and we are happy because the water is no longer boiling out of the pot. But the fire is still on, and after a while the water starts boiling again. And so, we add water again, and again the boiling stops. We can keep adding cool water for a long time, but at a certain moment the pot is full and there is no more room for additional water. But this is not a solution, because if we really want to address this problem once and for all we need to lower the flame of the stove. Then we need to understand why water boils, and it is not enough to know that cold water cools down hot water. Therefore, if we really want to solve in a definitive manner the problems of mind (which represents all the problems connected to our existence as individuals), we need to turn to the nature of mind.

Venice, April 30, 1983
Morning session

FIRST ROUND TABLE
Professor Monaco, Professor Donato, Doctor Trogawa Rinpoche, Doctor Lobsang Drolma, Doctor Tenzin Chödrak, Doctor Luigi Vitiello

Moderator: Professor Giorgio Monaco

Barrie Simmons: Professor Giorgio Monaco, professor of internal surgery at the University of Roma and director of the Center for Traditional Asian Medicine at ISMEO in Roma, will speak and moderate this morning's round table. We have with us also Doctor Luigi Vitiello, an Italian doctor who studied Tibetan medicine and has written a book, on sale here, presenting and introducing Tibetan medicine. I will let them take the floor together with this morning's presenters.

Giorgio Monaco: I thank our friend Simmons for his introduction. Let us now immediately turn to the people who will engage in our conversation. We will begin with our round table participants and then we will engage with some selected questions in order to draw some conclusions on all that has been presented so far. It is actually quite important to try and understand and modify a part of our attitude toward Tibetan medicine. As the host and out of chivalry, I would like to invite to sit here at my right first of all Lobsang Droma, the first female doctor to officially graduate in Tibet in 1956. She studied in Kyidrong province, as her father and grandfather's pupil, for fifteen years. In 1960 she moved to Nepal, and then on to Dharamsala, where at His Holiness' the Dalai Lama's request, she directed the Center for Tibetan Medicine since 1972, and where she also runs her own clinic. In my view, on top of her scientific knowledge and professional qualifications, the doctor possesses a special warmth – a particularly positive vibe.

Next, I would like to invite Doctor Trogawa Rinpoche, a Tibetan doctor renowned in Sikkim, who studied in Lhasa and was for nine years a student of the great master Nyerongsha Amchi La. Afterwards he went back to Lingbu, his Nyingmapa monastery, where he was in charge of fifty students. Equipped with the general preparation taught in Tibetan medical schools, is open to all questions and will facilitate any conversation at a general level. I would like also to invite to join us Professor Donato, the director of the Institute for Technologies Applied to Cultural Heritage of the National Research Council, who is a world authority in the field of fragrances and cosmetics. Professor Donato will serve as an example of a Western scientist who decided – and we shall hear why – to deal with the difficult field of Asian medicine. I would also like to have with us Doctor Moscatelli, the secretary of our Center, in his role as translator and expert of Tibetan culture.

As it is often said in conference introductions that go on forever, I "shall be brief," and will try not to intrude upon a world we came here to listen to, the Tibetan world introduced in a global fashion to us in this wonderful gathering, in a way that has opened us to the mindset of Tibetan medicine. I would like to simply note our difficulty in understanding this world, and the process, and often the ordeals, that we have to face to try and comprehend traditional Tibetan medicine. In my view, a fundamental concept we need to underscore from the beginning in this universe is the idea of the relationship between humans and environment preserved by Tibetan medicine. Thanks to our good fortune, we have with us Father Klasinsky who helped us formulate this idea in philosophical terms as the relationship between micro and macrocosm. I will remind you that medicine is always connected to the socio-cultural context in which it develops: unavoidably, each medical system is affected by the environment in which it is created and develops. This way all of humanity's history recognizes some basic fundamental steps such as magic-religious healing of the shamanic type. For instance, in pre-Buddhist Tibet the Bön period was characterized by a medical culture mostly based on magic-religious cures of the shamanic kind. The arrival of Buddhism in Tibet entailed an enormous experimentation, a promotion of culture that brought the collection of books and the blooming of great colleges, universities, institutions, and cultural legacies. Let us not forget that traditional Asian medicine has the great advantage, in comparison with other parts of the world, to belong to a literary culture. African practitioners, Philippine curanderos, as it is the case for many other cultures around the world, rely on oral cultures that often get lost with those who practice them. In Asia, instead, we have books, texts, universities, and this is very important. Therefore, we are dealing with a living ancient culture.

A third point I would like to raise deals with modern medicine. In the West, the so-called scientific, modern medicine has made huge progress and has solved certain problems –think only of diagnostic science, of MRIs, ultrasounds, scans, all incredibly modern and non-violent tools that respect the individual's person, and are therefore most acceptable and non-invasive. Unfortunately, however, modern medicine has followed a one-way, one-directional trajectory. And so, we find ourselves in a cul-de-sac: if we follow the logic of this framework, at the end we diagnose patients with our machines without even seeing the persons: we de-humanize the relationship of doctor-patient. Here, instead, we find the richness of Tibetan medicine, which sees the whole picture, and holds a global vision of human beings, because it cannot ignore that they are part of a general system. And our friends have taught us, also graphically, how to reconstruct this universe through those wonderful compositions – the mandalas. In them we see how Tibetans simultaneously evoke by analogy the East, the color green, and Spring: they embrace all the categories of concepts connected to general laws.

And this is the richness of this vision, of this approach. And I, at least for now, would like to stop on this clarification: the diversity lies in the approach – in seeing things in a different way. As we move through our conversation, listening to our friends and to others, we will see what other ideas are necessary to integrate these two kinds of medicines.

My presence in the National Council for Research at ISMEO served also to promote a general conversation about traditional Asian medical systems that I believe is important to briefly introduce to you, in my introduction, through succinct slides so that you may, today, in the context of your meeting with Tibetan medicine jot down a few thoughts, a few ideas, that based on our experience are very important as a result of our collaboration. If I could please have the slides, I will comment on each of them briefly, as they are self-explicatory

SLIDE 1. Traditional medicine, of which Tibetan medicine is an example, is the medicine that develops following the format of a tradition – I have noticed that the public is particularly sensitive to this concept, namely, Tradition with the capital T, which means many things: it is the combination of the knowledge about health and sickness derived from the cultural tradition of a people. Please note this concept of health and illness. Regrettably you know that still today, in the definition of the World Health Organization, health is the lack of sickness. Consider how incomplete this idea is, how mutilated, lacking in all that wonderful knowledge that in Tibetan medicine instead defines health as the harmony of many functions of our body with many other laws of general importance, such as the cyclical, seasonal ones, and so on.

SLIDE 2. So, what are the peculiarities of traditional medicine in general, as well as those of Tibetan medicine? It consists of the global vision of a human being inside the ecological system. We Western doctors see a person as a disassembled machine (whose anatomy we received from the German school and whose workings were taught to us by some following research in physiology after the war): it is nothing more or less than a body – something that works as a mammal. The discourse of Tibetan medicine is much richer: if we take for granted that there is a body, but also something else, this is where we have to investigate, because if we disturb this "something more," illness and therefore an imbalance may arise. This concept is very important because it allows us to research and recognize traditional systems in the context of the WHO. It is not expensive. But luckily for us, this time just because something is not expensive does not mean that it is not worth a lot, quite the contrary, and we shall see why.

SLIDE 3. What are the characteristics of traditional medicine worth preserving? Traditional medicine is part of popular culture. You will find remedies that date to the Bön period, that depend on the Buddhist doctrinal vision, all the theory that goes from the five elements to the three humors of human physiology, all tightly connected to the unique Tibetan culture. Not only this, it has already been demonstrated that – and you can see this yourselves – that there are many therapeutic systems not yet tested, that have not yet undergone a so called scientific demonstration, that nonetheless give proven results and are effective in treating certain illnesses. Traditional medicine, if it is handed down, ensures the respect of a people's cultural heritage. I will not linger and explain which contribution Tibet has made to mankind as a whole. For us it is also a reservoir of ideas for scientific research because, in the immense natural park nature is and this incredibly articulated practice, there are studies that can lead not only to new medications, new remedies – a fact that is not so interesting to us – but that can also help to discard old views and bring us new ones.

SLIDE 4 How can we utilize traditional medicine? We have just explained how: upholding truly effective therapies, looking for new medications, and promoting research. I had already outlined these ideas earlier.

SLIDE 5. This point seems really important to me because you who are interested in Tibetan medicine must keep in mind its dangers and limits. First of all, we must understand our Tibetan colleagues. We start from different principles. If we hold on to our belief system, this will remain a conversation between deaf people. For this reason, our cooperation must include a lot of humility in accepting the other culture, but also great learning because we need to be able to assimilate the other culture without implanting dangers. The Western person who goes Oriental cuts a very sad figure, just as the Eastern person who loses their cultural identity. We also have the heavy hand of industry that, in finding truly effective medication, brutalizes its active principle together with the usage meant for it in its country of origin. The different concepts of health and sickness must also shape preventative medicine, because it is clear that Tibetan medicine is founded upon the observation and conservation of natural laws that require much more attention to the health situation than we normally give, and we do not do enough to assess whether a medication that can temporarily bring relief, improvement of a certain symptom, will eventually cause damage, and here we can think of the institutions represented by Doctor Donato, for instance.

You will recall that in ancient Greek *pharmacos* means both poison and medication, and all depends on how and when, and in which doses, it is administered. In this sense, Tibetans are better experts than we are because they administer medications in a very specific fashion, which means not because of the active principle medicine may contain, but mostly for the influence that that medication has on that particular patient in that particular moment in their energetic physiology. I would rather not speak to this last issue because, if I am here, it is precisely to destroy the professional jealousy that arises when two cultures face off. I want to say that in our missions among Tibetan people, with our Tibetan friends, I have never encountered a situation in which I could detect rigidity on either side, because the two cultures faced off with humility and steadfastness. What is serious, truly damaging and bothersome, is a "half culture," which means being arrogant. If you meet a person who thinks differently from you and that sees the other side of the coin, you can truly find a middle ground.

SLIDE 6. Another slide that can complete this concept of mine, that is, the utilization of traditional medicine. This reflects a bit what we have done: finding the operating hubs – universities, clinics – cataloging therapies and probable active mechanisms. Here lies our contact, our conference, and the opportunity to be with the practitioners and do cultural exchange, after which we can also move on to this promotional application. What I said could be represented by the last slide. This is the improvement that can come from our collaboration, because using a system that already exists, we can make progress in the basic knowledge promoting research and also deepen our knowledge of illness.

SLIDE 7. How do we look at one another? The slightly chubby figure on the left is me, and the others are the children we met in Nepal for the last mission to study Tibetan medicine. I would like to conclude this first introduction with the question: "How do we, as East and West, look at each other?" That is the reality: I, on one side, as an individual, and on the other the East, with all those eyes.

I do not want to end this speech with my words, but with those of someone who is very important in the history of research: he said that very often the solution of a scientific problem lies, more than in instruments and mathematical methodology, in the possibility of looking at the problem from another angle, with new eyes. A scientific problem is often solved because one can see the other side of the coin. This entails a wonderful and authentic adventure in science. This is the meaning of words once spoken by Albert Einstein, and I believe it can become the light that guides our future collaboration with the Tibetan people.[10]

Our next speaker is Doctor Lobsang Drolma, who will speak about her experience and general principles and will also give explanations and clarifications not just about her activity as a doctor but also as a scientific researcher, which brought her to international attention for her push for the contraceptive pill of which you all have heard. I invite our colleague Lobsang Drolma to speak and to enlighten us with her knowledge.

Apologies, Lobsang Drolma just informed me that she will not present, as she prefers to answer to questions directly. We appreciate

10   The exact quote is "The mere formulation of a problem is far more often essential than its solution, which may be merely a matter of mathematical or experimental skill. To raise new questions, new possibilities, to regard old problems from a new angle requires creative imagination and marks real advances in science." It appears in: Albert Einstein, Léopold Infeld, *The Evolution of Physics* (London: Cambridge University Press, 1938), p. 92.

her gesture that, I believe, is a demonstration of tolerance and great openness. Let us see if Doctor Trogawa Rinpoche would like to speak.

Apologies, Lobsang Drolma just informed me that she will not present, as she prefers to answer to questions directly. We appreciate her gesture that, I believe, is a demonstration of tolerance and great openness. Let us see if Doctor Trogawa Rinpoche would like to speak.

Trogawa Rinpoche

We, as beings of the physical world, live in an environment made up by the five elements and are always involved with this world. We are in this world because we basically do not understand our true condition. This lack of understanding is our primary ignorance that is the primary cause of our basic irrational movements. This leads us to enter the physical world through the combined characteristics of our parents' blood [egg] and semen respectively. At the beginning, consciousness takes form on a merely nominal level: form, as an identifiable object, manifests at a very primitive level. Then, gradually it develops, and what develops basically are the senses. The development of the senses activates the contact with one's surroundings: this contact in turn produces the natural reaction of sensation. Sensation has a natural connection with desire, which in turn produces the inclination to attachment. As a result of this attachment to one's environment there is, as a consequence, the process of existence's becoming which is the process through which we evolve because we traverse the process of birth, and consequently, of progressive aging until death in the life of the three spheres of existence.

The root of all this is our basic ignorance. The reason why we undergo all kinds of experiences and suffering is due to this fundamental ignorance. In this life we also experience happiness, but it is ephemeral, passing, not definitive happiness. This process of existence does not really happen; it is rather a sort of dream. Due to our ignorance, however, we do not understand its dream-like nature, and existence appears real to us. We see many things in this dream-existence, and we think and feel in terms of friends and foes. What is damaging, or potentially so, we consider a foe, and what can benefit us, a friend. In this fashion, due to the attachment of the ego to our situation, we always put ourselves in difficult situations in our search for favorable conditions and our flight from unfavorable ones. All the circumstances to which we relate in this manner, choosing a few and rejecting others, are fundamentally unreal: the benefits we can gain and the expenses we can avoid are equally unreal.

The body we inhabit is our dream, and passages [channels] and winds [prana] structure it. Regardless of whether we are ill or healthy, in our body we have five kinds of winds and many channels through which the winds flow, but we will not talk about this now. Our body is made by five elements, and we live in a world made by five elements, and we get sick when these are not balanced. If the elements are not in balance, we must do something to bring them back to their natural balance, using medicine, diet, or changing our habits. In the majority of the cultures of ancient Asia we find the same concept of the five elements.

As far as medicines are concerned, I advise using the most natural products possible, meaning minerals, plants, and things that one can find easily in nature. When I say to use material that can be found in nature to re-balance the condition of the elements, I am not just talking about Tibetan medicine, but also about classic medicine in general. This holds true for both East and West: we can find in any environment the plants and natural substances necessary to re-balance the elements of the people who live in that environment. Our world and our personality are our individual dream: it is only a dream. There is nothing real in it, but for now it is our dream; it is where we are. If for the length of our dream we can live together in harmony and happily, this is a good thing; if we can avoid harming others and based on our circumstances act on behalf of others, this is very good. I hope you will remember this, and we can talk more about it later on. Thank you.

Moderator

This is a powerful message coming from that world we all love and that reveals great mental clarity. When truth emerges, you see that all conferences are magical moments in which the voice of a speaker, whose name we may not even recall, says things that belong to everybody. It is like a butterfly fluttering about: the ones who catch it for themselves ruin it, but if the butterfly is free to fly about, it is truly something that belongs to everyone, like the words of Doctor Trogawa Rinpoche that have come right after my attempt to clarify how things are. And here are our different approaches; his words, which engage emotionality and the psyche, cause only irritation in a misguided Western doctor. In his concise presentation, instead, you have witnessed the constant interchange between psyche, body, and adaptation. He spoke about natural medicine, which is the medicine that grows with the same general rules of life.

Our fantastic translator rendered humors with "airs:" you are all already experts in these matters, but in case you were not, the three humors are not meant here as air, phlegm, and bile in the chemical and physical sense of the word. Rather, they express general laws that have not yet been proven by the so-called official Western science but that in truth rule the world. Air is the expansion of the universe, the general movement that complements our planetary situation after the Big Bang; Bile is Fire, the chemical and metabolic changes in the universe and our body; whereas Phlegm is the general law – still unproven – that attracts and keeps together all the planets preventing them from dashing away in an erratic manner, and that we find in an identical fashion in the law of human physiology. Because Air – expansion – is nothing other than, for instance, peristalsis, according to Tibetan medicine, meaning the movement of the intestine, the heartbeat... Have you ever asked a Western doctor: "Why does my heart beat?" [His answer would be, most likely, that it is] because of the nervous system. Fine, who controls it? Well, it is automatic. Of course, it is automatic: it is connected to one of these universal laws, to a law with universal implications, still unproven,

but that the Tibetan mind knows perfectly. And here lie the differences
we were discussing just now and the challenge in approaching them.
Allow me to keep this conversation going a while longer along
the lines of the parallel study of these two medical traditions I carried
out, for the sake of the exchange in which we must engage in order to
understand one another. We have heard Doctor Trogawa give us the
structure, the general laws we could call them, of the five elements
and the three humors that are the foundation of all physiology. Now
allow me to ask now Doctor Donato, given his research, in his highly
qualified institution, of Eastern and Tibetan perfumes and incenses,
what drove him to this subject, and why he chose not to speak in the
Western scientific language, using a new language instead.

Giuseppe Donato

Frankly, I do not speak any language, and always prefer to listen. If
you wish, I belong to the dying species of listeners. Apart from not
having the gift of eloquence, I am a chemist, and thus the only thing I
can do is to tell you briefly about my experiences. As Professor Monaco mentioned just now, an experience I have concluded only few days
ago, which I displayed in an exhibit in Lugano and that will presently
travel to the States, deals with the reconstitution of certain perfumes,
better yet, of certain ancient ointments, and in particular Eastern ointments. It was an experience of experimental archeology, which is, as
you know, the attempt to reproduce through experiments and conditions as close as possible to those of the epoch [under consideration]
instruments, objects, and all that was necessary for survival.

Why this specific research on perfumes and ointments? First of all
because it is a research I like, it amused me, and I decided to undertake
it. I am not joking, because our research, to be truly valid, must be a
source of enjoyment and entertainment for us. This is the basis. I do not
want to linger on scientific research and so on, but I believe that this is
a very important matter: we must always put our passion in [research],
otherwise we will never be able to conclude anything. It will always be

something temporary. I recall a quote by Immanuel Kant: "If culture is the sail, passion is the wind." If we have no passion in what we do (and I am talking about the field of research), even if we have thousands of meters of sail [at our disposal], it will remain inert without the wind of passion, and we will not make any advance.

The research to which I devoted myself was born precisely from the need to study a problem that interested all of us, meaning the various ways and measures with which each civilization responded to its instinctive aesthetic needs. This was the start for the research, and we ended up with quite something else. Of course, the beginning entailed a serious, in-depth, and accurate bibliographical study of ancient texts in search of substances, plants, and all that could put us on the right track. For me it was a process of becoming one with what I studied. I would call it a journey of exploration in which, on the basis of ancient recipes, I personally rebuilt a personal alchemical laboratory. Basically, I did what the comparative study of religions does, in the sense that I reproduced the alchemical journey of the reconstruction of perfume according to antiquity, and today, knowing how a modern perfume is created, I am able to compare the two. As my work got under way, I realized perfume was something more than a flavorful substance: it was, it is, something connected to the living past world, I would say, because I realized through all I read in various documents that perfume – like color, music – is an experiential vehicle, an experience that moves in the depth of the subject, of the subject's unconscious. It is a symbol, and therefore a very effective tool to connect the external environment with the inner one.

My last, but for me the most, important consideration given my training is that it is exactly for this certain influence on mankind that perfume – and I am speaking about perfume, the odorous substance, and not about contemporary fragrances, which are on two totally different levels – can be used as a healing substance (I am not calling it medication) to alleviate various psychological, emotional, and also physical situations, because all of its components are pharmaceutical substances. According to one of the most modern and contemporary currents of thought, traditional medicine – about which I will not speak as I am here to listen and not to speak about either medicine or pharmacology – is an alternative therapeutic system to modern medicine. No, it is not an alternative system, rather, it is the attempt to understand the natural means humans have at their disposal to adapt to their environment. Research allowed us to see that almost all ancient perfumes were used as medications, and this is why I aim to study them still and to continue this research in the pharmaceutical context. Ancient perfumes were not only the expression of aesthetic taste, but also the expression of the environment in which these substances were inserted.

One of the most advanced recent acquisitions on the examination of the ancient world is the re-evaluation of a basic idea common to all of the philosophical and scientific doctrines of the past, especially the Eastern ones, namely, the lasting bond between macro and microcosm, meaning the constant interdependence between human physiology and the general laws of the universe. The vision of humans emerging from modern Western biology represents the unavoidable result of the loss of the symbolic knowledge of nature by today's people. This synchronization with the cosmos and with natural laws is the great wealth of traditional doctrines, especially Eastern ones, precisely because they have not neglected the fact that humans are part of nature and that, therefore, they are constantly in touch with the phenomena that surround them. The adaptation of living beings to this resonance between received input and adequate response finds in the five senses their fundamental vehicles.

In the exchange between humans and biosphere, sight, smell, and hearing especially represent the symbols at the basis of the phenomenon of life. Therefore, it is no cause for surprise that perfumes, colors, and sounds, since ancient times, have not only played a role in rituals, but they themselves were adopted as healing systems in their own right. It goes without saying that shallow information engenders shallow outcomes, as evidenced in the message of the visual sign of the street light: the red light immediately conveys the sensation of danger, it makes you stop if the information is perceived at a certain level. But if one can move beyond, red means something else. It means blood, violence: the [semantic] field can expand considerably. I would like to stop here. In summary, what I did was a rather rigorous scientific research, if I may say so myself, but on the basis of philosophical ideas.

Moderator

I believe that you will have listened with great interest to this learned but passionate presentation by Doctor Donato, which we have enjoyed. He proffers a much more generous vision than the one that prevails in our universities. Professor Donato is very rigorous when it comes to Western methodology, but also very open to the implications raised by Doctor Trogawa Rinpoche. This energetic physiology, these principles, these general laws govern also human beings, and are at the foundation of the Tibetan diagnosis of health and illness. This diagnosis happens also through pulse examination, together with anamnesis and urine analysis. I now would like to ask Doctor Lobsang Drolma to answer a related question from our audience.

Question: Based on what we have heard in these past few days, a pulse variation may manifest also in a healthy person. It is indeed possible to encounter a pulse that is not characteristic of the season one is experiencing at a particular junction. This can have two meanings, at least based on what I understood: it could mean that something is about to happen in the social environment of the person, meaning among siblings, in their family, or to other people connected to that particular person, and this is the meaning of the prognostication that we can conduct through pulse-taking. Alternatively, it could mean that there is something, some organ in that person that could develop an illness. I would like to ask how we can discern one case from the other.

Lobsang Drolma

If a person is not healthy, or is sick, the characteristic of the disorder manifests in the pulse. The pulse of a healthy person beats five times during a complete breath (inhalation and exhalation) of the doctor. So, if we have about 70 to 72 beats per minute, a person is healthy. We learn from the pulse if a person is healthy or unhealthy. If we feel an irregular pulse that does not correspond to that of a healthy person, almost certainly that person is sick: we cannot encounter a pulse indicating illness in someone that is healthy. There is nothing fictional in pulse examination: even in these days we took the pulses of various people and all the doctors present were able to identify the symptoms of the patients. Whereas Western medicine uses lots of machinery to diagnose illnesses, it may seem strange that we can have people who can make diagnoses with few instruments – six fingers – but Tibetan medicine is very ancient and has developed this diagnostic system. We have many instructions in this regard, some derived from ancient texts and other particular ones on the subtle distinctions between the various pulses, differences doctors learn through experience and that they transmit to one another. The doctor applies a higher form of knowledge when they examine the pulse. It is important for the doctor not to have a *lung* disorder because this could alter their sensibility and would not allow them to identify the various qualities of the pulse in an appropriate manner.

Moderator

Some questions, like the one raised by our colleague just now, are framed in a very specialized way, and therefore I skipped the first part, which dealt with the differences between the Tibetan and the Chinese pulses. It is undoubtedly an interesting question, which, however, does not allow everyone to benefit from the exchange with Doctor Lobsang Drolma, and therefore can be answered right after the roundtable through a private conversation with her. I would rather give preference to broad questions that can be of interest to everyone. I would then like to bring Doctor Lobsang Drolma's attention to this question about cancer in Tibetan medicine.

Question: Doctor, could you characterize for us the types of success-fully treated cancer and illustrate their differences? Cancer is an in-dustrial disease, at least in our areas. Which factors, in particular, can cause this? Have Tibetan doctors noticed an increase in cancer in their people in the diaspora, and if so, how have they interpreted it?

Lobsang Drolma

We cannot categorically state that cancer is an industrial disease. There are many and various causes that can engender it, and in any case the majority of tumors are caused by industrial pollution, smoke, and var-ious substances spread in the environment. Cancer, however, can be caused also by other factors. As I mentioned in an earlier presentation, breast cancer can be caused by excessive stimuli or constrictions. It would take a long time, however, to go over in detail all of the various types of tumors, since cancer can manifest in various parts of the body, for each of which there exist multiple triggering factors. I will there-fore examine one kind of tumor, namely, uterine cancer, and I will analyze it from the point of view of Tibetan medicine.

One of the possible causes of uterine cancer is the interruption of the menses. In my view, however, one of the main causes is abortion, which is very common nowadays. When they carry out an abortion, doctors use instruments that touch the inner organs, and this can trigger uterine cancer. Tumors may result also from C-sections. Also certain sexual practices can cause uterine cancer: some positions, as well as some unconventional sexual practices, make it more likely to manifest.

How do uterine tumors develop? There is a primary channel in the uterus that begins to swell. The body naturally carries microbes and par-asites within it, and a certain kind of parasite is drawn to the swelling in the uterine channel and penetrates it. This disturbs the balance between white blood and red blood, and this imbalance contributes to further increase the swelling. At this juncture, the symptom of constant loss of menstrual blood appears, and one can detect the illness in the face of the woman whose complexion loses its natural luminosity; hair begins to fall; abdominal pains manifest; and there is constant loss of white yellowish fluid.

In Tibetan medicine, we treat this illness with an infusion to dilute in water to flush the uterus. We prescribe three specific kinds of medication and a vaginal ointment. A few weeks after the beginning of the treatment, we prescribe another medication to apply on the abdomen in the area corresponding to the uterus. Uterine cancer can be cured in about two months. After the cure has succeeded, further treatment is necessary to ensure the menses return to normal. After having changed the medications, we also apply cauterization. The modality of applying fire, and also the usage of the golden needle, be it the standard or the silver one, depends on the specific characteristics of the disease. In the Tantras, we also have mantras to cure disease, and the faith of the patient in the practice and the capacity of the healer have to work together to work successfully. This relationship is like a hook and a noose: a hook can catch a noose, and draw it in, but if there is no noose – i.e., the patient's trust in the practice – there is nothing for the hook to catch, and the cure has no effect. The doctor must also have the capacity to carry out ritual cures. They must have recited the mantra of the Medicine Buddha, and they must have the capacity of the Medicine Buddha. If they do not have this capacity, it is as if there is a noose but no hook, and without the hook there is no way to catch the noose. In short, there is no need to worry about cancer if one has a good doctor, and if there is a way to cure the disease.

Moderator

We thank Doctor Lobsang Drolma for introducing all of these ideas. Since we are running out of time, we will ask a question that would deserve a whole conference in and of itself.

Question: Doctor Mario Liotti would like to ask Doctor Trogawa Rinpoche something more about the relationship between the three humors and the five elements, and in particular how the latter influence the former.

Trogawa Rinpoche

Five elements make up our body, and at the same time we also have the three humors, namely, Air, Bile, and Phlegm, which are not independent but tightly interconnected. Space is the element that pervades the other four. In this context, we need to consider, aside from the body, also mind. The elements are the basic material the body is made of. The three humors derive from mind: air rises from desire, bile from anger, and phlegm from ignorance or lack of awareness. Regardless of whether we are healthy or ill, we possess these three factors that derive from the three emotional qualities of mind. When we are well, these three humors are balanced. An emotional imbalance or a disturbance in one of the fundamental emotions will cause an imbalance of one or more primary humors. This will disturb the humors and the elements, causing an illness. The illness that follows the imbalance of the three humors can arise due to diet, habits, and behavior.

We have six tastes in food: sweet, sour, pungent, bitter, salty, and hot. We find them in various combinations, and each has an effect on Air, Bile, and Phlegm. These effects, in turn, can also cause the loss of their natural balance. These six tastes have eight different qualities, and from them we derive the tree secondary effects. The same holds true for actions. There is a connection between the various actions and the conditions of the humors. Therefore, as far as health is concerned, we want humors to be in balance. The wrong diet can potentially imbalance the humors and produce illness. To follow a good diet is one of the main factors for health.

Moderator

Our gratitude for this truly concise explanation that included general principles, physiology, as well as preventative measures. This is the culture with which we must engage, to which we need to relate. In conclusion, before the break between our round table and the next, I would like to invite Doctor Vitiello to speak, as a colleague who organized this event and as an expert in traditional medicine. We would like to hear his Western voice speak on the subject of medicine.

Luigi Vitiello

I would just like to offer a very short epiphany about ways to perceive nature that I had listening to all the teachers in these exchanges we have had. It seems to me that there can be two fundamental ways to perceive nature: either as raw energy, so to speak, to control with our own intelligence, as it were, or as something that is already perfect in and of itself, and that can be a teaching for us in a variety of ways. It looks like in the West we have always wanted to follow the first point of view. In other words, we have chosen to tame nature. We have obtained results in so doing, and interesting ones to boot, but that have cost us a great deal of effort. In the East, on the contrary, people have chosen to learn how to better understand and harmonize with nature's energy. In this fashion, they have obtained equally brilliant, and at time even better, results, without the energetic waste that we have experienced in the West. If humankind will in general be able to harmonize with nature, I believe that we will succeed in better reuniting with our real dimension because we are part of nature.

Moderator

We thank Doctor Lobsang Drolma and Doctor Trogawa Rinpoche for their contributions. I will not draw any conclusion now, because the second roundtable moderated by Doctor Simmons will keep building on these concepts later this afternoon. I believe that the best way to call to an end this session, which I have had the honor to preside, is to sincerely applaud in the spirit of the collaboration and tolerance taught to us by Tibetan people, the two translators whose names I do not know, but who, through their work, patience, and capacity, have allowed this conversation to take place.

SECOND ROUND TABLE
Professor Namkhai Norbu, Doctor Tenzin Chödrak,
Doctor Carlos Ramos

Moderator: Professor Barrie Simmons

Let us begin with our roundtable, which is not only the conclusion of today's gathering, but also, in a way, the summation of our conference, the first international symposium on Tibetan medicine, and hopefully not the last. We have already received various questions from the audience, and Professor Namkhai Norbu, Professor Tenzin Chödrak, and Professor Carlos Ramos, our conference's director, will take turns in answering them. I would like to apologize in advance to those whose questions will not be answered due to time constraints. We are also struggling with the translation process, because our translators will have to leave at a certain juncture, on top of which some important guests need to go away too, and so it is not easy to keep everything under control. For those who are interested and have the possibility to join us, there will be a follow up of this event in Arcidosso. For some there may also be the chance to have short private conversations on technical aspects that most likely will not be answered during this session.

We have a question here that goes back to the topic of cancer, already discussed this morning, as well as the other day in Professor

Namkhai Norbu's presentation. It is a comment on the fact that in Tibetan medicine the usage of the term "cancer" does not exactly correspond to that we find in Western medicine. The incurable cancers Western doctors have referred to are not necessarily the same inflammatory diseases Tibetan doctors have mentioned. And this can also be extended as well to other pathologies present in the modern world and are incurable for Western science as explained by the American colleague raising this question, who now asks for Professor Norbu's feedback.

Professor Namkhai Norbu

The other day I explained in a very general way what we mean by cancer, and I mentioned that, according to Tibetan medicine, it is not so easy to cure. I also explained a principle, namely that the Tibetan way to envision an illness rarely corresponds to the view-point of a Western doctor. In my view, this is a very important principle. On this basis, I explained that in the system of Tibetan medicine there are various kinds of cancer. I also heard Doctor Lobsang refer to this principle this morning. I am not at all saying that Tibetan medicine is a miracle cure, or that it can heal these diseases – it would be an exaggeration. There is no guarantee. I simply meant to say that Tibetan medicine has a way of seeing and working that keeps the existence of the individual in mind. The individual has a material body and a mind, and these two aspects are connected to energy.

I have explained this point on various occasions. It is very important for Western medicine to understand this aspect. Many people have told me, also in private, that Western doctors have a difficult time applying Tibetan medicine, and this holds true also for cancer. I honestly do not believe that it is impossible to apply it. The issue is rather the human limitations that I believe doctors need to overcome. For me, when we face a patient whose only concern is to get better, it does not matter whether a doctor is Tibetan, Chinese, Japanese, Indian, Western, or someone else, because it is not the doctor's title that will save the patient's life. The doctor saves a life the moment he or she enters the condition of the sick person and works with the patient, and this aspect is often missing.

I am sorry to say this, but if we do not understand this point, it makes no sense to speak about medicine for days on end. We hold our conference, speak with expert Tibetan doctors, with the hope that it will be also useful in the West, particularly for specialists. Many work with specific issues like cancer: people all over the world are fighting against it and trying to learn more about it, so why not deepen [our knowledge of] the view point of Tibetan doctors about this disease? We cannot argue that something difficult cannot be applied [simply] because there is a problem to overcome. In Tibetan medicine when we speak of an incurable illness or patient, we are not necessarily talking about cancer; we can die as a result of other illnesses that become incurable. Disease, however, can be healed when we understand it from the get go and know how to deal with it, meaning, that the doctor understands the patient's condition and the patient understands the doctor's work. There must be cooperation between them.

The principle discussed in Tibetan medicine is the understanding of our energy and of the material body. The body is connected through energy to the mind that thinks and creates problems. These are the aspects we have explored and discussed, and I have not much to add. The other day we said that there is a way to work with breathing. If we do not understand it, it doesn't seem like it makes much sense, but if we do, we understand that humans live by breathing; and that breathing is connected to energy; and that through breathing it is possible to guide energy. This knowledge exists also in traditional Chinese medicine.

You know very well how many explanations exist about acupuncture, for instance, and there are also many in Tibetan medicine on moxa and other therapies.

I heard some participants say that they would like to learn something concrete in this conference, but it is not easy. I can tell you that there is a therapy called moxa, but the most we can do here is to explain its function, we cannot hold a course in a few days, because medicine requires years of study and a lot of experience. And we can explain how mantras work, and how to intervene on the function of energy especially in relation to the illness of cancer, whose character is called lanyen, which means that cancer is connected to the provocations of outside energy through which this illness develops. We need therefore a specific way to work on it, and we have it in Tibetan medicine: it is in other words possible to intervene on these aspects, and there are many methods to do so. If a doctor is interested to learn more about this topic, my words will not suffice; they are simply examples. But you can learn more, and there are many things that can be done also in the future, hopefully. Why? Because a doctor's objective is to solve the problem. The problem of cancer exists, it is under everyone's eyes. I truly hope that our conference will be meaningful and helpful to all of human kind.

Moderator

We thank Professor Norbu. Cancer is one of humanity's greatest problems. I would like to now ask one of the most renowned Tibetan doctors to illustrate which are, in his opinion, its causes and to tell us some of his experiences in the treatment of this disease. I believe that this is important, so that we may perhaps be able to find a way to alleviate all of this suffering.

Doctor Tenzin Chödrak

In Tibetan, we use the word *tren* for the disease Westerners call cancer. How does this disease generally arise? It manifests in the body through an alteration of the blood and spreads to the various full organs like the heart, kidneys, lungs, and to the empty organs like the stomach, intestine, the colon, as well as to the blood, bones, marrow, and so on. It was not as widespread in the past as it is today, and the cause behind the increase of cancer depends on various conditions, like the increase in industrial pollution, behavior or life-style, the use of many alcoholic beverages, and certain foods. Today's situation is very different from the past, and this new situation causes the increase in cancer cases.

When there is a malfunction of *lung* or the humor Air, some cells begin to harden and to disturb the organs and other parts of the body: it is in this way that a tumor develops. When the process of cellular thickening begins, the entire body starts being altered by it. The conditions which cause this hardening and the *lung* malfunction are disparate. Among them we find worries and mental unhappiness, which lead to a *lung* disturbance that in turn engenders the rising of the illness. Another factor is large consumption of certain aliments, like beef. Another kind of tumor manifests when we drink too many sugared beverages. The combination of external factors (like the increase of factories and environmental pollution) with internal factors (like diet, behavior, and mental agitation) creates the conditions that lead to the illness, which can manifest in any part of the body: the colon, the stomach, or in any other organ.

For many years in India we did not have the *tsothal rilbu* pill, of which Professor Tsarong showed the preparation yesterday, but recently we have begun to prepare it. It is an effective medication for the treatment of certain tumors, like that of the kidneys, the bladder, and the bones. After a correct diagnosis, we administer it to the patient who improves within one, two, or three months, and who can later go in remission. For example, I treated cases of breast cancer that were in remission and then later returned. In the West doctors diagnose about six months of life in this situation, but my patients lived one year and a half. I also treated tumors of the nose: after administering medicine, the patient got better, so the treatment was effective. The pills we talked about contain many metals, like silver, copper, and gold. In the ancient texts of Tibetan medicine many medications are prescribed for treating cancer, but today we cannot use them because of the difficulty in preparing them: when we are able to prepare a few of them and test them for a certain period, we will prove their effectiveness in treating tumors. In the treatment of breast cancer, for instance, we also use moxa treatments. Compresses, made of various ingredients, are applied all around the breast, then we cover the breast with oil to keep it warm, and based on the reaction we see we can understand whether we can treat the tumor.

Many kinds of cancer develop along the seven constituents of the body, the five vital organs, and the six empty organs. Some may be caused by mind in various vital organs, or by excessive consumption of beef or alcohol, or by an excess of sugar or chemical substances. We describe fifty-two of them in our manuscripts. They can also be caused by inflammations.

Moderator

We have a question about bone diseases, especially those present since birth or genetic ones, and about treatments and cures one can carry out.

Tsarong Jigme

I am not a doctor, and I do not practice medicine, so I think it is more appropriate to ask Doctor Tenzin Chödrak these questions, as he is a practitioner of this profession and has great experience, and is the best person for clinical questions. I am simply an evangelist of sorts for Tibetan medicine and work so that people will become aware of the worth of this tradition: what interests me is not connected with the clinical aspect.

Doctor Tenzin Chödrak

One type of bone disease manifests as a result of living in humid places and being in excessive contact with water, as well as of eating food that is too acidic. In these conditions, *lung* becomes unbalanced and creates these problems: bones start manifesting various diseases as a result of lung's malfunction. External and internal conditions – and external conditions here mean, as we have just said, cold, humidity, contact with water, whereas the internal conditions are acidic food, i.e. diet, and an unhappy mind full of worries – combine and cause the rise of bone disease. Other bone illnesses come from issues with the digestive system, for example from food that is not digested well because the stomach lacks heat. In this case nourishing substances that are not assimilated well through the process that creates the seven bodily constituents cause bone illnesses as well. Another factor that can result in bone disease comes from nervous issues that affect bones as they spread around. An aggravating factor comes from problems with blood vessels: if blood does not flow properly, it affects the nerves and engenders bone disease. In terms of treatment, bone disease does not respond well to medication. But the pill whose preparation you saw demonstrated in yesterday's slides has proven effective in its treatment.

Then we have TB. This, as well as *chuser*, serum or lymph, can cause a torsion in the vertebrae, like the thirteenth and the fourteenth.[11] As treatments we use *ngulchu rinchen chogye*, and also cauterization, generally carried out with a golden instrument or also with moxa. When the vertebrae are completely rotated, it is very difficult, but if we catch it at the beginning it is possible to set them back in their place. Six hundred years ago in the tantras of Tibetan medicine it was said that there was going to be a time in which chemical agents and factories would grow and that, at that time, these diseases would spread enormously. External conditions in which chemical agents and pollution exist seem positive because they bring affluence, but there are other consequences. Thus, since both the body and external phenomena are made up of the five elements, there is a relationship between the body and the external environment. When external elements are manipulated and then assimilated in the body, or they enter on contact with the body, this relationship between external and internal elements causes damage.

In terms of the body, we have diet and behavior, medicine and therapies. The most important factors are diet and behavior: if we do not pay attention to them, treatment with medicine and therapies is very difficult.

Moderator

---

11   "Lymphatic disorders (*chu ser kyi nad*) are illnesses related to lymph or serum. Lymph (*chu ser*) refers to the sticky fluid located primarily below the skin and in the joints." In Chögyal Namkhai Norbu, *Healing with Fire*, Part One, note 20, Shang Shung Publications, 2011.

I would like to stress that we now have enough questions, aside from the ones previously submitted in writing, and requests for another conference. Thankfully we will have another gathering in Arcidosso, so those able to attend it will have the chance to explore many of these issues in depth and receive answers. As for today, we only have enough time for one last question for Professor Namkhai Norbu: many people would like more clarifications about the way in which Tibetan medicine treats mental and nervous illnesses.

Professor Namkhai Norbu

Tibetan medicine treats illness both with medication and with behavioral and dietary recommendations, as well as with various kinds of specific therapies like moxa, acupuncture, and so on. Mental illnesses are considered to be tightly connected with the function of energy, so it is not only medicine that deals with them, but also the teachings, like yoga and Tantrism, which have developed a great knowledge of the energy of the individual, of its connection with breathing, and the way in which to utilize breathing to coordinate vital energy.

The treatment of mental illness does not apply exclusively to madness: the disturbance can simply arise from a state of confusion or nervousness. We all understand, for example, nervousness, because we all have a material body and the function of energy. When the function of energy is not correct, when it is not in perfect condition, we are confused. When the disturbance is very strong, we can call it madness, but in lighter forms it can manifest as confusion, or as shutting down, without the capacity to communicate with others, or it can also transform into a feeling of extreme sadness. And the list could go on.

Everybody experiences moments like this, and consequently Tibetan medicine advices to learn to coordinate one's own energy through breathing. In Sanskrit energy is called *prana*, in Japanese *ki*, in Chinese *qi*, in Tibetan *lung*, but even if the words are different, the reality is the same, we are always talking about our vital energy. All mental disturbances are related to this factor. Therefore, as I always say, understanding mental disturbances is strictly connected to our understanding of the interrelation of body, energy, and mind. If we do not understand the nature and function of energy, we do not understand the causes and remedies of mental illnesses. If you are interested in this topic, you can profit from our upcoming meeting in Arcidosso where these matters will be discussed extensively. I hope this way you will be able to become free of any doubt.

Moderator

This morning I tried to suggest that, sooner or later, each of us could make an appointment with one's own deep self and that the communication between our busy and conditioned self and our deepest identity and reality could not be that simple. But when this encounter, this appointment, takes place, it requires work and attention, and possesses great worth. From a certain perspective, I think this is what has happened in these days. It is the meeting of a part in each of us with another part, the inner self, the encounter between a knowledge grown in the depth, in conditions of relative isolation and peace, that now becomes part of our common heritage, and our breathless and often awkward Western way to understand and not understand deep messages. Before calling our meeting to an end, I would like to ask Doctor Carlos Ramos, director of this conference, and its main motor and animator, to whom we owe great gratitude for making it possible for this gathering to take place, to make a few concluding remarks.

Doctor Carlos Ramos

I would like first of all to pay homage to my Master. Then, I would like to say something implicit in the presentations of the Tibetan doctors and teachers who have spoken in these days, and explicit in private conversations, namely that people who want to heal others must first of all heal themselves, observe themselves, and perfect themselves. If they do not do this, they cannot heal others.

I would also like to reflect on what we have been doing here in Venice. We have in some sense made history. About one year and a half ago we organizers had the idea of gathering the Tibetan doctors to meet with them through an exchange of ideas. Then we acted on our intent. Also, the Tibetan doctors, when they learned about the conference, had the intention of coming here and acted on it. And you as well, when you received our brochures, took action. Now, in these days, we have reached the third stage, the stage of satisfaction. Intent, action, and satisfaction are three extremely important elements of our conduct. What does this mean? That our intent, our action, and our satisfaction belong to the history of Tibet, to the history of Venice, and also to the individual history of each one of us. And so, it is a past event. We always want to do something, we act on it, and then become part of history, but most of the time we are not aware of it. And death comes while we are still thinking about making history.

How can we make history and live with awareness? I would say that the only way consists in observing oneself, what happens inside of us, how our being can integrate with what is happening, with all people. For instance, if I succeed in integrating with my Master, with his wisdom, I can see through his eyes, and he can see through my eyes. Not only that. I can see through the eyes of his teacher, and they can see through my eyes. In this condition wisdom and clarity become concrete, and then our behavior is complete. I hope that this idea, implicit in the words of the Tibetan doctors, can help us to take back our Western roots, because it is not as if we do not have this teaching. We have this teaching, and it is a rather good one. And thanks to the Tibetan doctors in this moment we are always aware of our roots. I would like to thank my Master and the Tibetan masters who have brought life to this event of awareness, which may aid in our growth and maturity and that may help us doctors to lessen the suffering of others, because we cannot eliminate the suffering of others without working on ourselves first.

Before coming to the end, I would like to thank first of all the Cini Foundation and its staff, who have allowed us all to work in the best circumstances. I would like to thank the registration staff, the translators, and all the people in the office who worked so that this conference could take place. Last but not least, I thank all the public and cultural associations that made this encounter possible, this bridge that, as Tsarong Jigme said, will allow us to unite our technical and material knowledge with practice to arrive to the inner knowledge Tibetans possess.

Tsarong Jigme

On behalf of the Tibetan doctors, I would like to thank everyone present here, especially the organizers of the Dzogchen Community and Professor Namkhai Norbu. We hope to have planted at least one seed, the hope that someone will keep studying and supporting this medical tradition that I personally believe to be very important and endowed with great potential to help people. This is the main objective. We are not here to say that Tibetan medicine is the only medical system, there are many: the doctor's duty is to know them, so that they can provide the best medical possible to the patient. We have been very happy to take part in these proceedings. Thank you again.

Arcidosso

Arcidosso, May 2–7, 1983

214

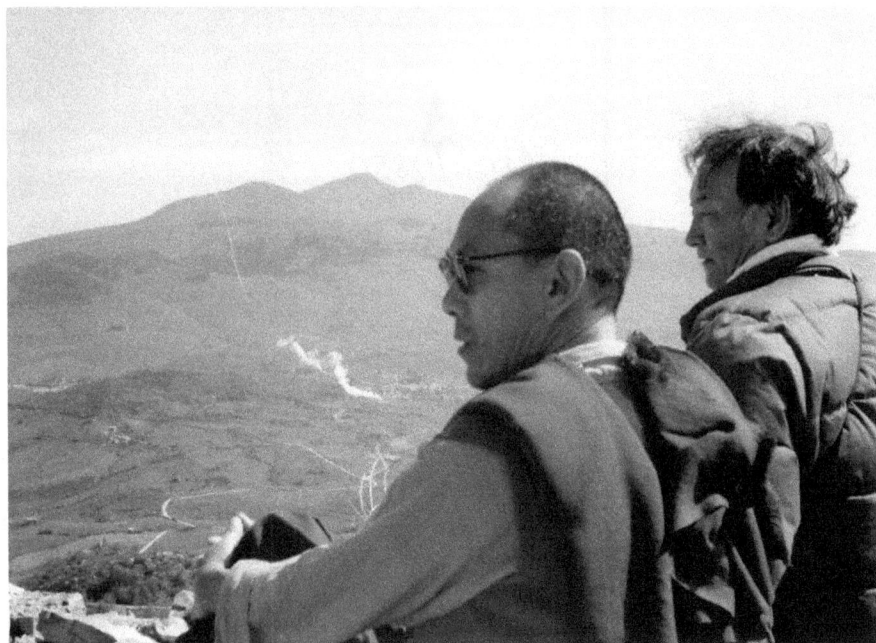

Professor Namkhai Norbu and Trogawa Rinpoche on Mount Labro
(Photo by Carlos Ramos)

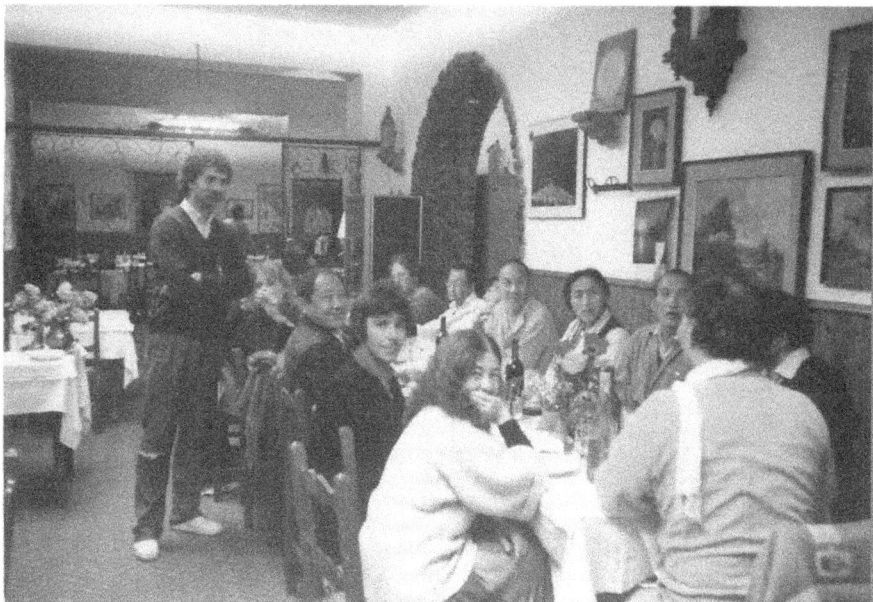

Social gathering at the end of the conference in Arcidosso
(Photo by Luigi Vitiello)

Arcidosso, May 2, 1983

INAUGURATION
*Professor Namkhai Norbu; Paolo Rosa Salva,
architect; Marcello Bianchini, J.D.; Doctor
Marcello Ramacciotti*

Moderator: Paolo Rosa Salva

My task today is to declare open here, in Arcidosso, the second part of
the First International conference of Tibetan Medicine, whose first in-
stallment came to a close last Saturday in Venice. I would like to recall
that in Venice the proceedings were particularly interesting and very
well attended. While the first session was more theoretically oriented,
this one in Arcidosso will have a more technical and applied aspect
with direct demonstrations by our guests, the doctors, for the Western
doctors or the audience part of this gathering.

I must once more stress here, just as I did in Venice, the part played
by the local associations in Veneto and Toscana in organizing this
conference. The municipality of Venice, the Province of Venice, and
the Region of Veneto, the Region of Toscana, the Province of Grosseto,
the Mountain Community of Mount Amiata, and the municipality of
Arcidosso were involved in sponsoring and contributing to this event.
In general, in Italy, local administrations have stepped up their role in
facilitating and increasing cultural exchanges among different ethnic
and national groups, and are promoting this development in a climate

of friendship and mutual collaborations among different groups. In this context, we find, next to local groups, numerous Italian cultural foundations, such as the Cini Foundation, which hosted the Venetian side of this conference together with the Querini Stampalia Foundation, the Ligabue Foundation, the W.N. Badmajew Stiftung (pro-Tibet) Foundation – Zurich , together with the Procuratoria of San Marco in Venice.

Having thus described the general picture in which our meeting takes place, I believe that we can now invite the mayor of Arcidosso, Marcello Bianchini, to speak, so that he may convey the greetings of the citizens of Arcidosso to the participants.

Marcello Bianchini

I was in Venice to greet the conference participants, and I will of course do the same here in Arcidosso, as it behooves our township in its role of host to greet and thank the organizers of a conference of considerable cultural significance. In Venice I had the opportunity to explain the reasons behind the Comune of Arcidosso's participation, as promoter and host – meaning in terms of the administration that hosts this conference – and I noticed the importance of the fact that through cultural exchanges, in this case about a very important topic like medicine, we are able to deepen the meaning of the friendship among populations and peoples, and to reach, through dialogue, great objectives in the peaceful cohabitation at the global level. Therefore, no matter what judgement may be passed on this kind of initiative, by the operators in the specific sector we are dealing with, or by observers who are simply curious and interested in general, I believe that this initiative carries the deep significance I have just mentioned. We should also consider that a conference like this, aside from having a general cultural relevance, creates the chance to exchange ideas in the specific area we are dealing with. As a matter of fact, I think that no science has ever reached, in and of itself, such level of perfection and completion to the point of being able to dismiss what another science that developed in another country or is practiced by another population may have said, done, practiced, and invented.

Consequently, even from this point of view, I think that the most serene and constructive attitude is one that excludes subservience or condescension and is based on openness and dialogue. For this reason, we have joined this enterprise, and let us not forget that here in Arcidosso we have the Dzogchen Community, led by Professor Namkhai Norbu, which has great success both in terms of participation and cultural interest and is promoting cultural and human initiatives of great worth. Of course, as I speak these words, I believe that we will try on our end of things, within the sphere of our competences, to ensure that the connections now happening in Arcidosso, and in the area of Mount Amiata more generally, between the Dzogchen Community and our citizens will happen in such a way to enable as much as possible moments of understanding and mutual sharing. The speaker who preceded me thanked all the local institutions that contributed to the organization of the conference both as promoters and as sponsors. Going by the number and the quality of the participating associations, we can deduce that the conference has undoubtedly been very successful. I must note that, aside from the illustrious names listed in the conference program, we have here among us also the second secretary attached to the Embassy of the People's Republic of China, Lu Ho Chin Piao, with apologies if I am not pronouncing his name correctly. Therefore, such an authoritative presence from the Chinese Embassy indicates that this great country and great people are interested in this initiative.

I thus thank the participants, and I hope that this event will enjoy success and an engaged attention and that everyone will enjoy, on our mountain, a stay worthy of the hospitality we want to offer. I will now invite the moderator to speak.

Moderator

I thank the Mayor of Arcidosso, and invite the president of the Comunita' Montana of Mount Amiata, Doctor Marcello Ramacciotti, to speak.

Marcello Ramacciotti

It is my honor to welcome all the participants on behalf of the administration and the board of the Comunita' Montana, and to wish you all a pleasant stay on Mount Amiata. We are especially thankful to all the illustrious scholars and representatives of prestigious associations and the organizers of this First International Conference of Tibetan Medicine that we are pleased to host in our area. I feel that we need to especially recognize Professor Namkhai Norbu and his collaborators, who we have already had the chance to meet during their residence on Monte Labro. I also think that we must acknowledge the meaningful presence of the second secretary of the Embassy of the People's Republic of China, that indicates the particular interest around this topic and an issue that generates great interest on the part of the press and the cultural forces in our countries at an international level. This meeting engenders great interest as well because for the first time it puts us in touch and in exchange with scholars and representatives of a civilization, a culture, a history that for us encloses and expresses fascination and mystery. In our day and age, characterized by a frantic development of scientific research and technology, we also feel the need not to lose, I dare say, to recover, new human values of brotherhood and solidarity that exalts human creativity and affirm peace and cooperation among peoples. The aim of this conference offers a reflection on a culture, knowledge, and expression that are specific to the Far East, but the space, the resonance, and the conclusions that, I am sure, will emerge from our gathering, so qualified and representative, will not fail to elicit, even in our society, various reflections on the vision of human beings. Our land preserves and expresses cultures and traditions that push us – in terms of our thoughts, initiative, and research – to affirm more and more broadly human values and solidarity between humans and peoples. Even for this idea that animates us, we find particularly meaningful this gathering that puts forth its contents in a cosmopolitan dimension.

Please accept, ladies and gentlemen gathered here, my wish for a productive experience and a pleasant stay in a land that knows how to give and receive human warmth and solidarity.

Moderator

I thank also Doctor Marcello Ramacciotti for his introduction and his greetings, and I now invite Doctor Franco Vianello who represents here in Arcidosso the Alderman for Culture of the Provincial Administration of Venice, to speak.

Franco Vianello, Alderman for Culture in Venice

Mine will be a short greeting on behalf of the President of the Cabinet of Culture of the Province of Venice, with our wishes for success to all of those who have contributed to the organization of this conference. It is important to stress that, beyond the narrow sphere of legal competence, the provincial administrative office of Health and Assistance felt compelled to adhere and contribute to the organization of this event both because of its great interest and the implications in historical, cultural, philosophical, and political terms, that an exchange of ideas involves – not only within the context of Tibetan medicine, which always raises great interest since it is an unknown world in terms of its methods and the underlying philosophy in the medical practice itself – and because of surely broader reasons, such as a meeting of civilizations, a need to communicate that must find a larger development in our time. We need, as a matter of fact, to confront and learn new styles, modalities, and practices of living in terms of the medical and therapeutic aspects as well as of the complex of communal and civilized living at an international level, giving in return our experiences. Thank you.

Moderator

Having heard the greetings of the representatives of local associations, I invite Doctor Tsarong Jigme to speak on behalf of our guest, the Tibetan doctors.

Tsarong Jigme

Dear Mayor, honored citizens of Arcidosso, ladies and gentlemen, I would like to thank, on behalf of the Tibetan people and of the doctors in attendance here, the Italian cultural organizations for sponsoring with such great enthusiasm the First International Conference of Tibetan Medicine, held first in Venice and now here in Arcidosso. After our eventful schedule in Venice, I personally feel that in the course of the next six days we will be able to engage in even more depth with our medical experience, thanks to the experience acquired in Venice, and to the fact that we have here a natural mountain scenery. I believe that it is meaningful that we mentioned that Tibetan medicine is one of the most neglected among the four great medical traditions of mankind. At the same time, we will explain its fundamental tendencies in academic and practical terms, and we will also demonstrate some of our methods and specific techniques, with the hope to raise your interest so that the doctors will seriously turn to this tradition in order to contribute to the improvement of living for the benefit of human beings. Thank you.

Moderator

I thank Doctor Jigme, and also our kind translator, and I invite Professor Namkhai Norbu to speak on behalf of the Dzogchen Community.

Namkhai Norbu

I would like to first of all thank all those who organized and sponsored this meeting, part of which we have already conducted in Venice. I would like also to thank all the participants and the Tibetan doctors. I am not thanking myself, even if I am Tibetan and a doctor, because, in a certain way, even if I am originally Tibetan, I am also an Italian citizen, since I have lived in this country for many years. I believe that this conference is very meaningful and important not only for Tibetan culture, but also because it is something very concrete. As a matter of fact, medicine is connected to the culture of each country, and yet it is most of all connected to the condition of each individual. From birth until death, we live facing many problems that never cease, and medicine is one of the best ways to solve them. We are not dealing with Western or Eastern problems, but everyone's problems that affect all of human kind. Generally, we have limitations connected to one country, culture, its specificity, there are many limits, but I believe that medicine is a very lively means for all human kind.

As Doctor Tsarong Jigme said, Tibetan medicine is a concrete asset that we need to learn and practice. I do not mean as something limited to the culture of Tibet, rather as something that has authentic value for all human beings. Keeping this in mind, let us use it to benefit all human kind. We are trying to collaborate with Western doctors at this level: if there is something positive, we need to reciprocally understand it, learn it, and put it to use. This meeting has given us a chance of truly meaningful exchange, and so I would like to thank all those people that committed to its realization, and I hope that everything will go well and that we will reach a positive outcome.

Moderator

I thank Professor Norbu, and I now invite to speak Doctor Ramos, Director of the Centro Medico di Psicologia Applicata in Venice, who organized this conference in collaboration with the Dzogchen Community.

Carlos Ramos

I would like first of all to pay homage to my teacher. A year and a half ago, when we began organizing this conference, our Master shared with us a few auspicious words. They say that such words, having come true, have great power. I would like to read them to you because the conference in Venice, and its follow-up here, are their realization: "Victory in all directions!"

Why Tibetan medicine? What does it have to do with us? You can find the answer to these questions in the image you will find inside your

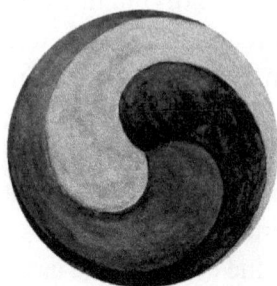

Figure 5. The gakyil

conference folders: it is a *gakyil,* a sphere of three colors – blue, red, and yellow – which represent the three conditions of humans, namely, mind, energy, and body. These three conditions cannot be separated: when mind separates from body, disease manifests; when body separates from energy, disease manifests, and death comes. Thus, this is the central issue. This is the vision that we, our forefathers, our ancestors had of humans, and that, in a certain manner, we have lost in the last few centuries.

What do we want? We do not want to become Tibetans, because I cannot become Tibetan: this is my culture, this is my condition, this is my environment. And therefore, from the Tibetans I can perhaps learn awareness – the instruments to see myself. I will give you an example. In his book, Professor Namkhai Norbu talks about birth and death, of how a baby is born, of how, beginning with energy, two cells unite until they form a new being. This is not knowledge that Professor Norbu just acquired, it is a twelve-hundred-years-old tradition that has been transmitted to the present day. When did we discover the existence of sperm and eggs? Only at the end of the nineteenth century. But in Lhasa there are thangkas, paintings, and drawings created more than six hundred years ago that show the entire process of fetal growth. What does this mean? That they are more intelligent than we are? No, it does not, but perhaps it means something else that we have not realized, namely, that there are different ways to get to knowledge. And these ways are the important ways to travel on in this moment.

Through this microphone, for example, we can amplify voice in a way everyone can hear it; and if we put an outside speaker, people will be able to hear it also outside. Thus, this is the projection towards the outside, towards matter, towards nature. This is a path, a walkway towards knowledge, collecting information that nature can give us. But there is also another way, the inner way. If I protect myself, if I know myself, if I am truly aware of my energy, my mind, my body, I can have knowledge of my entire body, and simultaneously know what is out there, matter. Tibetans have this knowledge. And my wish is that our culture may integrate these principles with the knowledge of our technology.

The question is not to disarm technology – quite the opposite. I believe that technology is important; it is one of human kind's conquests, a way to eliminate the many problems human kind experiences. Technology without humanity, technology without this global vision can lead to the destruction of the entire human kind. In this very moment, satellites and airplanes full of atomic bombs are flying over our heads. This is the negative product of technology. There is a positive one as well, however: through scientific research and agriculture we have eliminated a lot of diseases and we have increased the production of food and nourishment to feed the world. Therefore, it is possible to ride technology, as it were. How can we manage it? Only through the awareness that technology must serve human kind and not the other way around. The only way to achieve this is to return to the earlier example represented by the drawing of the gakyil: we must recall we have a mind, and our mind must be aware of itself; of the body, and the body must be aware of itself; and of energy, and energy must be aware of itself. In this moment, in these conditions, we can integrate what is external – that which is matter, nature – with our inner part and come to this unity.

What is all this for? It serves a very simple purpose, as Professor Norbu said: to alleviate suffering. Because we doctors have one role, that is, to eliminate suffering. We can eliminate suffering when a disease manifests, but we can also prevent it. We can lessen pain, but in order to do so we must be aware of these three functions, of these three components that form all of our human kind. The program here in Arcidosso will differ from that in Venice in that it will allow us to get to know a bit better how the Tibetan doctors, the Tibetan masters, see, observe, and cure people. We therefore have created a program that will allow us to hear them present their principles in the morning, and to see them interact with patients through practical demonstrations in the afternoon. Consequently, for the entire duration of the conference, we will hold every morning here in Arcidosso theoretical sessions, and in the afternoon, starting at four pm, we will have the practice sessions between doctors and patients. Simultaneously, for those interested, we will speak at the same time about nature of mind in Merigar.

Any question may be submitted in writing, and on Saturday, May Seventh, we will hold a meeting with all of the Tibetan doctors so that they may provide the answers. We arranged the conference in this fashion so that it is easier to group and answer various questions by topic. Before closing, I would like to thank the members of the Dzogchen community who have worked so hard to make this location into a welcoming place for us. I would like to thank the communities of Napoli, Roma, and Venice that have truly become the pillars of this entire event, and that through their hard work have created the foundations for it. Thank you.

Moderator

Now that we have heard from Professor Ramos, we can, I believe, call to a close the inauguration of the second stage of this conference of Tibetan medicine here in Arcidosso, and we will reconvene tomorrow morning in accordance to the schedule posted at the entrance. I invite everyone to partake of the refreshments in the lobby to wish us all success in our conference endeavors. Thank you, and good bye.

TROGAWA RINPOCHE
Mental Illness

The individual is made up of body, energy, and mind. Illness, even when it is physical, is always connected to mind, and thus spiritual teachings that can heal the illness alongside medication become fundamental. Accordingly, it is important to understand the nature of mind and find the natural state. Behavior and food, made up of the five elements, influence mind: physical illness, as a matter of fact, depends on the imbalance of the elements and the five *lung*s or airs. Diet therefore is important, just as the knowledge of the elements of which food is made, their heaviness. The lightness or imbalance of *lung* in an individual is caused by the constant use of light food devoid of substance, constant exposure to wind, mental stress, hemorrhages, insomnia, logorrhea, exhaustion, and anguish. In these conditions, we lose awareness of our actions and time. Hallucinations and fear, or paranoia, may follow, too, for instance, because of having personally lived a situation like war or for having listened tales about war.

Activities and food are governed by mind, which is in turn controlled by the *lung* of the body, which is in turn controlled by the channels in which energy flows and that irradiate throughout the entire body. How can a person become mentally ill? Madness can be sudden or we can have a progressive degradation that manifests through frequent yawning or boredom with everything, pain in the joints, decrease in sensorial perceptions with relative loss of hearing and sight, and alterations in taste and touch. As a cure, a few massage sessions are useful, combined with diet and behavior modification.

In a more advanced stage of the illness, we have symptoms like mental weakness, disturbed sleep, tinnitus, difficulty in opening and closing one's fingers, cough and phlegm in the throat at four o'clock in the morning, alterations in breathing, diarrhea, fear that others will speak badly about oneself, dry and rough tongue. In this situation, we must examine the urine, the pulse, and the tongue, and, aside from modifying diet and behavior, we need to administer medications, especially when *lung* is combined with other conditions.

Madness is the loss of the normal control of mind caused, usually, by a strong anger due to the fact that things are not going as we wish. Subsequently, aggression (*lung* pervades fire), suffering, shutting down, numbness, mental stupidity (*lung* pervades earth and water), and madness develops. As a cure, food must be very nourishing, the patient must be kept warm in a harmonious environment, and take walks outdoors. Furthermore, we must avoid judging the person and avoid making them feel under surveillance. You must keep in mind that strong light can be annoying because it influences the *lung* that runs in the channel of life localized at the top of the head, and thus closer to the nervous centers.

Mental illness can derive from a reaction to particular external situations, and, in this case, one must treat the person like a normal family member. Or it can be caused by internal factors, and then the doctor is the main player in healing and advising the patient.

The situation is worse when the person is uncomfortable everywhere, shows an aggressive or apathetic behavior. We need to be very sweet with these patients and administer medication to lower the strength of lung. There are forty-two different *lung*s associated with mental illness, but generally diet related to *lung* ailments prescribes avoiding fired and roasted food (whereas boiled food is great), coffee, sugar, wine and alcohol in general in excess, and pork.

In short, we must take our mind seriously. Disease is provoked by unhappiness with what one has. Thus, we need to be grateful and satisfied with everything we have and do. We should not force or compel our children in fabricated structures; they should study in a regular fashion, without pauses or explosions of over activity. We should apply ourselves in each activity with calm, regularity, and steadfastness, without worrying about what will happen, and do everything with awareness.

TENZIN CHÖDRAK
The Nature of Mind

Mind produces thoughts without ever ceasing its activity. But what is the origin of thoughts? If we analyze the question carefully we discover that it is not possible to find the origin of mind's movements: there is, in fact, nothing at all to discover because the essence of mind is emptiness.

Everything arises from emptiness, however: thoughts, phenomena, and our very self, which are all illusory experiences, like rainbows. We have projected an outside world, and the outside world projects onto our own mind. Since mind has no existence, all phenomena projected externally are empty of an independent nature: just like the dreams that arise continuously when we sleep, all that happens in our daily life has no independent reality.

On the other hand, all phenomena of samsara and nirvana are not separate from enlightened mind: they are not mind and are not separated from mind, and it is important to understand that, while they do not have a mind of their own, they manifest in a very concrete fashion. Even wisdom arises spontaneously from within itself, but it does not possess an objective existence that can be identified. Actually, not finding a self in mind is the most important discovery we can make, and we must understand it immediately, beyond any doubt. This is possible only through mind, and, in particular, thanks to the teaching and the direct contact with a Master.

Reaching the true vision of reality is very difficult, we need to accumulate merits and wisdom working on the meditation on divinities and mantra recitation. Working in this way with the energy of the deity – who we should not consider real, but like a reflection in a mirror⌐ – we are able to slowly free ourselves from the patterns and habits that entrap us.

Why must we accumulate merits and wisdom? To purify the karma that we have matured. Deepening meditation, the process becomes clearer, but it is first of all necessary to pacify mind and then to meditate on our own self. Our mind is conditioned by attachments and identification. It is like a container full of dirty water: we need to learn to calm our mind before moving on to the meditation on ourselves. Initially it is useful to retreat to an isolated place. We sit comfortably, cross-legged, without tensions, with mouth slightly open, breathing normally and naturally, gazing at our nose tip or upwards, without following memories or thinking of the future or the present. We simply do nothing, and we leave our mind as is. When we leave it in its natural state without fixating on the three times [past, present, and future], thoughts will of course arise; we just need to be present and observe them. If we become aware of them in the very moment they arise, thoughts dissolve and self-liberate just like a snake that coils and uncoils itself.

Mind can be left in its natural condition; at the beginning it is best to meditate repeatedly for short periods. If we encounter problems with our breathing we need to exhale slowly imaging our mind leaving together with our breath. We apply in other words "vase breathing" that we can learn in Yantra Yoga. If we meditate for a long time, mind becomes light and hidden memories, buried in the unconscious, can resurface. As a matter of fact, during meditation, when mind is aware, "gross" thoughts may arise, as well as "thin" ones, of which it is difficult to take notice, like water that runs invisible underground.

In our daily life, it is important to refer to meditation without, however, becoming attached to it and to slowly return to normal activities without rushing in anything we do and without becoming distracted. If we learn to meditate, our behavior is more present and our mind purer, and we feel in harmony with ourselves and with the world.

LOBSANG DROLMA
The Nature of Mind

The self is the cause of transmigration in the three realms of existence. But where is it? Inside the body, or outside of it? Where does our idea that we have a self come from? When and where does it disappear? If the self is not part of the body, is it something totally different from it? How can we define it? Does it have a form and a color? And if so, which ones? Or is it without form or color? Why are we convinced that the self truly exists? We must reflect deeply on the idea of the self. Is the person who begins an action the same one who completes it? Those among you who were thinking a short while ago, are you the same people who are thinking now?

If we consider any given action related to the body, speech, and mind, we can see that each time we make it, it turns out different. This means that nothing is real because everything changes and is impermanent. And again: let us consider our little finger, and let us imagine it breaking into pieces. Which part is its essence? Does it have an essence? It is important to discover our own self beginning with the three existences of body, speech, and mind, so as to comprehend the principle of emptiness. Any given object, for instance this table here, even if it possesses an apparent material reality is actually empty. This is the emptiness of form. We can continue to investigate and ask ourselves what emptiness is, what it resembles. And furthermore, we can ask ourselves if there is a difference between body and mind, like it is

234 ■ M<small>AN</small> – M<small>EDICINE</small> – S<small>OCIETY</small>

the case between the outside and the inside of a building; if mind dies, or not, and so on and so forth.

When we dream, we usually find ourselves somewhere else and we relive episodes from our past, or we anticipate future events. We have these experiences because we live in samsara, and our tendencies related to body, speech, and mind – good or bad as they may be – are connected to the experiences we have had in this life, or in previous ones. These basic tendencies depend on the attachment that creates desire, that is, the impulse to grasp and accumulate, whose origin is found in our senses. We depend on the outside because our senses are directed outwards, but we can turn them inwards, towards ourselves, without remaining passive towards them. This means to realize the potential of mind, an extraordinary opportunity that we have as human beings and that we should not lose. Wasting it is like pointing a finger towards the mirror, which turns against ourselves. This means that our karma depends only on us. What we are now is a product of our own selves – there is no determinism.

We are free, and our freedom consists of being able to realize what we look for. Our mind is free and pure from the beginning, but when it is distracted demonic aspects manifest. Like [it is the case with] a glass of muddy water, if we leave it still, the impurities will settle at the bottom of the glass and the water will become transparent. This means that we must first of all calm our mind. Mind is like the clear, open sky, which contains everything, but it is not easy to let it free: meditation can help to reach this level. When we reach it, this is meditation: in this sense, in Dzogchen, meditation is not meditation.

The state of meditation gives awareness, increases a state of well-being, cordiality, and happiness, and discharges emotions. It is necessary to find one's own path, one's own way to feel good, like the mountain that has its own dignity, which is not rigid but does not move.

May 6, 1983
Morning (First session)

NAMKHAI NORBU
Man, Medicine, and Society

You may have noticed that on the poster for our conference there is a figure that may look like either a man or a woman. It depicts Yuthog Yönten Gönpo the Elder, one of the most famous and important Tibetan doctors of the past, who we think lived towards the end of the seventh century CE. Tibetans consider this doctor a Master. I have personally met many masters, spiritual masters, that is. For instance, I spent five or six years in a college where we studied mainly Buddhist philosophy, but the master of our college was a great doctor under whom I studied for the first time the famous Four Tantras of Tibetan medicine.

Later on, I was on the border between China and Eastern Tibet, where I met another teacher who was very famous as a spiritual master, and not so much as a doctor, but who was, in truth, also a great doctor. I studied under him the Four Medical Tantras again. Lastly, I met the man who was for me one of the most important spiritual teachers. He was known as a doctor, and he often and mainly introduced himself as such. As a matter of fact, a teacher will manifest in different roles. At times, we can meet a teacher who will present himself as a doctor, or as a monk, or as the head of a monastery. Alternatively, we can meet doctors who are also yogis, practitioners; or doctors who will introduce themselves as normal people and live a normal lay life. The last teacher I mentioned was mostly this type of lay person, he was not a monk, but in truth he was one of the most important spiritual teachers of his time. This means that those who practice medicine must possess true knowledge.

Generally, we see human beings and medicine as subject and object, but we always need to understand the principle well. In Tibetan, the true meaning of men, medicine, is "benefit;" medicine, therefore, is something that benefits the individual. But in order to truly bring benefit, we must first of all understand the existence of individuals. Someone may have a physical problem, for example, a headache. But this headache may have a deeper cause: beyond the physical level there is always the individual's mind. A doctor must understand this fact in order to be able to heal through medicine. When we speak of medicine usually we mainly mean material things, especially in the Western world, where technology is very developed. For example, if someone asks their doctor for medication to get rid of a headache, the doctor may offer a more complete explanation, saying that perhaps a massage may help, or they may suggest a certain kind of diet to overcome the problem. But today many people are not satisfied with these remedies and will say that they do not have time to do those things, and they beg the doctor to prescribe an effective medication to quickly get rid of the pain. This is the current situation.

Eventually the doctor ends up satisfying the patient, enabling that attitude. Society depends on economy and circulation of money. If I, as doctor, prepare a medication that cures the deep root of the illness, but that does not have an immediate result, people most likely will not be interested in it; on the other hand, a medicine that makes pain immediately go away will be very successful. Everyone works a bit in this direction, so our knowledge decreases. Going back to the earlier example, if we get a headache, there must be a very precise reason: it could be bad digestion, a liver problem, a sinus infection; it could also be nerves – there could be multiple factors. Thus, we need to know how to work concretely with the existence of the individual and to understand if the problem depends on energy, mind, or simply is at the physical level.

Perhaps many people are getting tired of hearing every day Tibetan doctors speak about the cause of an illness, that is, of the three humors, lung, tripa, and peken, or, going more in depth, of the three passions, but this is a very precise and concrete principle. Even in the West people say, "Do not get angry, or you will ruin your liver!" It is the same principle. Passion is mostly connected to mind. The endless workings of mind slowly disturb energy, which in turn triggers disease at the physical level.

By medicine, we do not even mean that the doctor will make a kind of miracle to heal the patient: rather, the doctor has a certain knowledge of the condition of the individual, but complete remission can only happen through the collaboration of the patient. The individuals themselves must be interested in gaining certain knowledge: this is what we call awareness.

For instance, healing a disease is not just about taking a medication: one of the most important medicines is diet, what we usually eat and drink. Medicinal substances have a certain power, and generally we use those as well. But in the Western world there is a specific way to see things. For example, if you ask advice about diet in general, on what is good and what is harmful, perhaps a doctor specialized in macrobiotics will tell you that eating tomatoes is not good. But for Italians not eating tomatoes is a problem, because Italy produces tons of them! That is not exactly the principle: there is no food that is always beneficial, and another that is always harmful. For this reason, yesterday and over the past few days, the doctors have spoken about many different substances, of their worth, of the energy they possess, and so on. And they have also spoken of the way in which they use decoctions. Many know a medicinal plant, and they use it to make a decoction. Thinking that perhaps it is good for the liver, they harvest it and make a tea out of it. But this is not how medicine works. At times a specific decoction can be used for a specific problem, but there is no individual whose only organ is the liver, there are other organs, other functions. Something that we think is good for the liver; if taken excessively, will damage the heart. This principle is the fundamental basis of the diet.

Therefore, the explanation Doctor Jigme gave yesterday was very important. When we speak of pharmacology, we must consider the taste, energy, and quality of a substance. To truly know which substance will benefit us, first of all we must know ourselves, our condition: only then will we be able to assess what we need most. I believe that most of you have a book I wrote, *Birth, Life, and Death*.[12] In the last pages you will find a short analysis that can serve as an example, a list of foods used on a daily basis: I am not saying that eating a specific food is beneficial; rather, next to each item you will find three kinds of numbers that refer back to earlier tables. Each number gives a precise idea of the characteristic functions of the substance. Before this list, there is also a table that explains how we accumulate *lung*, *tripa*, and *peken*. If we read closely what causes their imbalance, we understand that in our diet all the substances that help to decrease them are positive for the individual. But it is not only a question of diet in general, another very important factor is conduct, behavior. For example, in the West it is very common that when people are tired because of their job, they will go and rest immediately after a very large meal. This is considered a normal thing. Nowadays also Tibetans in India have taken up this habit because in a warm climate, with a full stomach, one gets sleepy easily. Why does one get sleepy? It is a manifestation of *tripa*. The characteristic of sleep belongs to *peken*. To sleep in the afternoon disturbs *tripa*, bile. In Tibet, we never let a sick person sleep in the afternoon. In the case of certain diseases, to sleep in the afternoon immediately causes fever. There is an illness, called *nyenka*, in which the influence of negative forces that disturb an individual plays a role. One of the worst disturbances of this kind is caused by sleeping in the afternoon. One can think: "I always sleep in the afternoon, and nothing has ever happened to me." It is not for sure that the disease will manifest immediately, but once it does, it is there, and it is not positive.

Medicine in general helps us to live well, in an aware manner. For instance, people who have a *lung* tendency that is particularly strong do

---

12 Chögyal Namkhai Norbu, *Birth, Life, and Death*, Shang Shung Publications, 2008.

not usually sleep well at night. But if they start walking up and down, like many do, when they cannot sleep, after a while they will exchange night with day, and this is not going to help them. On the contrary, this will develop the *lung* even more. So, we have a whole series of structures and behavioral habits that can either help an illness develop or calm it down. There are many diseases, especially *peken* disturbances, that necessitate open air, luminous places, like the mountainside; with other diseases, instead, it is best to stay indoors, in the dark. This means that we cannot have fixed rules for the behavior either. The best thing is for the individuals to become a little bit aware about their own existence, which includes body, speech, and mind. This is very important: any teaching you will meet will always be based on these three considerations, just like any cure for illness must be based on this knowledge.

The physical body is connected to the entirety of our material dimension. We always apply this concrete knowledge, but we then have mind. Mind is not a material object that we can see and touch; thoughts, however, arise constantly, and we tend to follow them and to fall into reasoning. If you observe well and try to understand where thoughts come from, you will find nothing. Still, they keep arising without ceasing. In Buddhist philosophy, we say: "There is, but there isn't." Some say that this is just dialectics, but it is not like that. It is a real and concrete experience. When we say that there is not, it means that we cannot find anything that we can establish as object. And yet, even if we find nothing, we cannot say that there is nothing either, because many strange ideas keep arising. It is very simple: mind is like this.

For example, if we have a thought of hatred, and we follow it and develop it, rage and anger grow, and from these emotions actions ensue. If we observe well, all confusion comes from mind, not from the body. But what connection exists between body and the so-called mind? The connection, in our terminology, is called energy that in yoga we call *prana*, vital energy, and is connected to breathing. For this reason, in yoga it is said to train in breathing, which is considered one of the most important means to coordinate energy. In Chinese medicine prana is called *qi*; the Japanese, in Aikido, call it *ki*. In any case, the true meaning is that breathing is always connected to energy.

Any teaching, no matter what, is always introduced with three principles: to apply it, we first of all explain the position for the body, then the specific way of breathing, and finally the condition for the mind. Why do we always speak about these three principles, that is, body, speech, and mind? Because this is the condition of the individual. Even in medicine we must be extremely aware of these three aspects. If we do not have this knowledge, medicine becomes like an object through which we try and do something. With medicine, we do not mean the situation in which a doctor, in their study, examines a patient, prescribes some medication, and then the patient leaves: this is relative. The most important thing is to make the individual responsible. Doctors must have this understanding because they will always have to face sick people; if they do not have it, the patient will simply ask for medications to eliminate pain.

Western doctors, in meeting Tibetan medicine, ask first of all how to learn it. This is a rather difficult enterprise because, given that this medicine is written in Tibetan language, we must first of all to have a certain understanding of that language which, unfortunately, is not as widespread as English or other languages. Not only that, but there is no organization to teach it to foreigners. So, there are obvious obstacles in this sense. It is not easy to understand Tibetan medicine, but at the same time I am not saying it is impossible.

It is necessary first of all to understand what we mean by "Tibetan medicine" and its principles. We must, in other words, acquire an understanding of the existence of individuals. When we speak of a way to heal a disease or to conduct analyses, it means that we are entering a very specific field. Specific things can be learned slowly, they are not indispensable to Western doctors because Western medicine is for sure already quite developed. I am convinced that the great benefit Western doctors can take from Tibetan medicine is its way to conceive of human beings and of medicine itself. This does not entail changing or giving up on Western medicine and embracing another. Many people immediately put limitations saying "ours" and "yours." Others tend to build the stereotype of Tibetan medicine as spiritual, different from other medical traditions, and in so doing, they create problems between the Western tradition and the Tibetan one.

I personally do not see a conflict; rather, I believe that the fundamental point is to understand that we are all human beings and that we exist. Our being Western or Eastern people does not change a thing: a nervous Tibetan is no different from a nervous Westerner. What we need to understand is why a person is nervous, and what is the best way to overcome this nervousness. This is not so much related to nationality. Humans utilize their culture because that is the knowledge they possess. For instance, Western culture is very different from the Tibetan one. And we are not talking about the West in general: specifically, Italian culture, for example, is different from the English one. Accordingly, the knowledge of individuals depends on where they were born, how they were educated, how they grew up, and everyone finds it easier to use their own culture which they have experienced. But in order to utilize one's own culture, one needs to enter into the principle of knowledge: we each must become a bit aware of its meaning so that we will not find conflicts between cultures; rather, our knowledge will increase.

I will give you an example. Someone suffering from appendicitis, a very painful condition, may think that they do not want to undergo surgery, preferring natural medicine, and they want to use Tibetan medicine as a cure. So, this person will perhaps have to suffer for a long time, whereas it would be much easier for them to go to the hospital and have the appendix removed with one simple surgery. But someone refuses to have the surgery saying that today, in the modern world, everyone acts as if we were machines. In my opinion, this view is not correct, because we have situations in which surgery is necessary. Considering human beings just like machines whose parts can be replaced is not correct either, however. If human beings were only physical bodies, it would be easy to take out parts and put in new ones. But in many situations, we do not know how to connect them to energy, and then we can block many things. We need therefore to acquire a principle of knowledge and

242 ■ MAN – MEDICINE – SOCIETY

apply it as much as possible. If we have a certain understanding and knowledge, both Western and Tibetan medicine can truly be helpful and important. As I always say, medicine must help those who have problems and who want to overcome them. When someone has a problem, their first wish is to overcome it in any way possible: a doctor must keep this in mind quite clearly.

In Venice, I heard some doctors say that Tibetan doctors were explaining rather complex things, and they asked how they could apply them here. It is true, it is not easy to use such things, because Tibetan doctors have been studying for years, and explaining matters in two or three days, or even in one week, can not solve everything. Other interested people asked where they could deepen their knowledge of Tibetan medicine, explaining that they could not study it at their universities, where it is not taught, and that there are no Tibetan doctors who will be constantly on the road to teach courses. It is not easy, this is true. And yet, if we understand the principles, something can develop, one way or another. Thus, it seems to me that the main point is not to enter in a very detailed fashion in specific topics. In this conference, the most important thing for us is to understand the point of view of Tibetan medicine. This is the key to know it, and it may also be a key to increase awareness in our daily life.

By medicine we mean neither a theoretical study conducted on books nor medications. As we have already said, Tibetan medicine comprises three parts: medications, behavior, and diet. Medications relate to two different issues, namely to strengthen the body in such a way that it continues to be healthy and to heal it when a physical disturbance has already occurred. The same holds true for behavior and diet: if we understand this point, we have a way to collaborate with our own selves.

This is why I think that the most important thing is to be aware. Awareness encompasses everything. I will give you an example. Usually we discuss all sorts of problems: a doctor will speak about the specific issues of a patient, or about health matters within a hospital, like the number of beds available, medications, and so on. All our efforts are directed towards the material dimension. This is the case not only with medicine, but with society in general. But the most important thing, in the end, are the individuals who make up society. What does society mean?

Society is formed by individuals. It is like when we speak about numbers. "Numbers" is a generic plural noun, but in a concrete way we must start to count from number one, and then we have two and three, and so on. If we did not have "one," we could not have "one hundred." It is therefore very important to understand one, rather than one hundred or one thousand. The number one is actually the awareness of the individual, otherwise all of society's problems we constantly talk about are false. The qualification of human beings is the capacity to reason and to understand. And if this is the case, society cannot be compared to a flock led by a shepherd. This means that we are the number one, every single one of us: I am part of society, also someone else is part of society, and thus many people together are called "society." Then I must be first of all aware of my existence, of having a physical body that is related to the entire material dimension. If I eat something that is not good, I will not feel well, and my physical body will be disturbed by it.

List of Invited Speakers[13]

1. Doctor Jampa Thinley, Director of the Lhasa Institute of Tibetan Medicine
2. Doctor Troru Tsenam, Director of Studies and Scientific Research in Tibetan Medicine in Lhasa
3. Doctor Tsarong Jigme Tsewang, Director of the Institute of Tibetan Medicine in Dharamsala
4. Doctor Trogawa Rinpoche, Sikkim's most famous Tibetan doctor
5. Doctor Sangyey Tenzin, Tibetan medical doctor in the Bön tradition
6. Doctor Ama Lobsang, Tibetan medical doctor in Dharamsala
7. Doctor Tenzin Chödrak, doctor for His Holiness the Dalai Lama, Dharamsala
8. Professor Namkhai Norbu, faculty member in the Istituto Universitario Orientale di Napoli

Organizers
Dzogchen Community
Medical Center of Applied Psychology, Venice

Sponsors

Veneto Region

Province of Venice

Municipality of Venice

---

13   Unfortunately, Doctors Thinley, Troru Tsenam, and Sangye Tenzin from Lhasa were unable to join the conference proceedings.

Professor Pio Filippani Ronconi, University of Naples Federico II
Professor Carlos Ramos, Dzogchen Community and Medical Center
of Applied Psychology, Venice

PERMANENT RESIDENT EXPERT
Professor Namkhai Norbu, University of Naples "L'Orientale"

ORGANIZING COMMITEE
Doctor Enrico Dell'Angelo, Rome

Doctor Andrea Dell'Angelo, Rome

Doctor Giacomella Orofino, Rome

Doctor Luigi Vitiello, Naples

Doctor Ana Maria Humeres, Venice

CONFERENCE DIRECTOR
Professor Carlos Ramos, Venice

GENERAL SECRETARY
Architect Paolo Rosa Salva, Venice

www.ingramcontent.com/pod-product-compliance
Lightning Source LLC
Chambersburg PA
CBHW022054210326
41519CB00054B/407